Gentle Y(

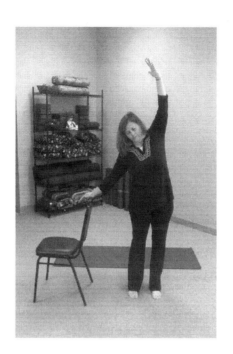

A Lifespan Yoga® Introduction

By
Beth Daugherty, M.S., M.A., E-RYT, RCYT

Gentle Yoga: A Lifespan Yoga Introduction

Dedicated to my students

Acknowledgements

I dedicated this to my students and they are the reason I wrote the book. I am so grateful I can get to know my students and they have trusted me enough to share their stories and challenges. This is what challenges me to refine my teaching and make it as practical and useful as possible. We are all students on the mat and in the world. Teachers are everywhere. This is so clear to me when I teach gentle yoga classes. Students are my inspiration. I also thank my husband and son for all their love, and support. Namaste.

Gentle Yoga Pose List

Gentle Introduction

Let's face it, yoga has left the ashram. Yoga studios are on every corner, yoga classes are on the gym schedule and now yoga breaks are common in schools, hospitals, churches and office conference rooms. Yoga pictures are a favorite background for TV commercials and yoga pants are a staple in the wardrobes of women who do not even like yoga. But what the heck is yoga? Is it an exercise program? A religion? A new way to meditate? Was it one thing a long time ago and a different thing now? It has changed, and continues to change, this practice we call yoga.

If you are new to the practice, you will be interested to know yoga is Dharmic tradition, not a religion, meaning the focus of the practice is on universal ethics like nonviolence. Many yogis around the globe see yoga more as a peaceful way of living than an exercise routine. Experts tell us yoga originated in India and that some elements of yoga predate Hinduism, Buddhism, Judaism, Islam, Christianity and other organized religions. Some of the traditional yoga practice is rooted in a time when people lived much closer to the rhythms of the earth and some of it is thoroughly modern. Yoga blossomed together with eastern religions, spread through the world and has grown to the popular activity it is today. It has endured into modern times as a self-development tool practiced by millions and was recently declared as popular as golf.

Almost every style of yoga in the west today is Hatha Yoga. Gentle yoga is a form of traditional hatha yoga. It is very slow and relaxing. In the way I learned and the way I teach, all the poses are modified to their most accessible form based on your body type, limitations, flexibility and strength. There is no expectation of sweating or of losing weight, although these things can happen, but there is the expectation of calming down a busy mind and reducing stress. When the most comfortable shape of a pose is found by a student, their body will relax. When the body relaxes, the mind can relax, stress melts away and from here meditation is more likely. There are physical benefits and biological changes with a gentle yoga practice. A calming of the central nervous system, lowered blood pressure, and increased circulation, flexibility and strength. Studies have found that regular practice can improve memory, reaction time, balance and coordination. There are also psychological benefits like increased focus and clarity, the reduction of pain and a heightened sense of peace. Gentle yoga promotes a noncompetitive environment which is psychologically different than many other environments we operate in.

Gentle yoga appeals to people who like a yoga style that is peaceful and easy to keep up with. The room is usually a comfortable temperature and the pace is slow. People with conditions such as ADHD, cancer, fibromyalgia, anxiety, multiple sclerosis, depression, OCD, arthritis and post traumatic or sensory disorders may attend this style of yoga class on the recommendation of their doctor. Especially when we add chairs and yoga props, the practice becomes accessible to many more people. In gentle yoga each pose will look different for each person because of the diversity of health, body shapes and sizes. In some traditions yoga was taught one teacher, one student. It was universally accepted each student was completely unique and each pose needed modifications for each individual. I like to teach from this tradition.

In 2010, I began this book a guide for my yoga students and teacher trainees, many of whom did not possess stereotypical "yoga bodies". In some cases, my students were battling serious health concerns such as cancer or chronic diseases, and were determined to find a gentle yoga practice because they were convinced it helped their healing dramatically. Students with pain, disabilities and special conditions are always looking for comfort in a pose, so I attempt to speak to them here. I have also had students who attended my yoga classes toward the end of their life, maybe learning poses for the very first time, and they have found great solace in this practice that helps us all face the inevitable.

This book is all about finding comfort and peace in the poses for the various stages of life. You will find I label the poses with the common English name and the Sanskrit name, fully aware that some teachers may use a different English name and never use Sanskrit. The Sanskrit pose names help yogis around the globe speak a common language. These names often come from stories of animals, gurus, sages, or gods and goddesses in ancient mythology. Like so many fables from around the world, these stories also have morals or lessons for adults and children alike, which I have noted in a few spots throughout the book. I also made up a few names myself! There is unlimited creativity in the yoga world. Those of you who are teachers will recognize the Sanskrit name of the pose, but don't be alarmed when you see I have adjusted the expression of the pose to a gentle form that works much better for many of my students. I have included pictures of myself and my family members doing some of these adjusted poses with help from chairs, the wall and yoga props.

My students know I am a big fan of the entire eight limb yoga system. I think this system is what makes yoga so accessible to people of all ages, stages, shapes and sizes. The first limb of yoga outlines how to get along with others in a civilized way. The second limb outlines personal disciplines for a healthy life. The third limb represents the physical poses or postures we practice for physical flexibility and strength. The fourth limb is physical in nature because it involves breathing techniques, but is also a doorway to the higher meditation practices in yoga. The last four limbs are also gateways to deeper and more profound meditation. Like climbing a tree, you can take your time with each limb and hang out on a branch one day and another branch another day.

My other books go into detail regarding the eight limbs of yoga, as well as the ethics, psychology, human development and meditation practices, so here I will just touch on some of these themes after the pose description. I include some common sense precautions about practicing each pose. At the bottom of each page, I include a little box where you can write down your thoughts about the pose or your progress. You can note the date and think about each pose individually. Do you like it? How does it make you feel? What are the thoughts circulating around in your mind as you do the pose? Yoga teachers may want to note other adjustments they find helpful or aspects of the pose they like to teach.

Gentle Standing Poses

Each yoga session usually begins with time set aside for centering, getting grounded, surrounding yourself with positive thoughts and setting an intention. Centering can be as simple as sitting in your most comfortable position, cross-legged, lotus pose or in a chair, taking a breath or two and remembering why you are practicing yoga. It is important to settle down and let go of outside distractions before you begin. All the thoughts about work or whatever is on your mind can be put aside for a time. The whole idea is to let go of these things to give yourself a little respite; all of your concerns will be waiting for you when you are finished.

What does get grounded mean? In my class, I encourage everyone to get grounded by feeling the place where their body parts touch the floor or chair where they are sitting. This is to become aware of where your body is in relation to the space around it and the physical support you have in different places as you feel the weight of your body. After getting grounded, I also like to imagine the space around the mat or chair as a bubble of positive energy to work in. This also brings your awareness to the control you can exercise over your space, even if it just a little mat or rug.

I like to have my students set an intention at the beginning of yoga practice. I usually offer them a moment to set an intention for their practice, their day, week, year or life. It can be as simple as "I intend to stay focused" or as grand as "I intend to create world peace". This reminds them of the reasons they practice and what they want for this moment and this life. It is a seed planted and the following practice will be like sunshine and water to encourage growth and development.

The set of poses presented in this first chapter are gentle standing and balance poses. In a gentle class, we move slowly and mindfully through a few of these poses, taking great care to stay safe, holding on to a chair or the wall if needed. After our beginning meditation these classes often begin with standing and balance poses to build strength for the more challenging seated poses. I have also included some fun facts here and there after the pose description.

Breathing techniques are an important part of yoga. The first three breathing patterns will sound familiar, but in yoga we distinguish them from each other. The first is a *Cleansing Breath*, which is a deep breath to reset your breathing patterns. I call this the *Mommy Breath* in Kids Yoga because all moms and kids know this sound. A mother is worn to a frazzle, nothing is going right, no one is listening to her or helping her and she stands at the kitchen stove, takes a deep breath and exhales a huge sigh. That is the perfect cleansing breath. Another basic breath is the *Resting Breath*, which is not really a technique but just a natural breath. I call this *Baby Breath* because like a baby resting in a crib the breath is natural and even. *Breath Awareness* is when the primary focus is on your breath. It is one of the foundations for all yoga. Begin by using your mind's eye to watch your breath go in and out of your nostrils. This is very important in yoga and teachers will always remind you to watch your breath.

As you move through the book, feel free to select which poses feel safe for you and pick and choose among them. You may want to spend some time getting comfortable with these poses, and each can be practiced at a few levels of difficulty so you can experiment, challenge yourself or back-off at any time. I include a few pictures for most poses so play around with the one you like or adjust it to fit your special conditions, body and health.

Mountain Pose (Tadasana)

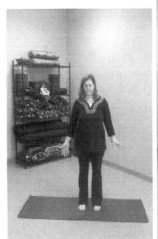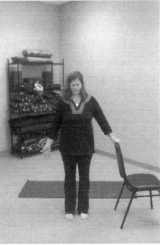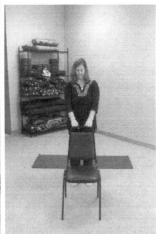

Mountain pose is a place where many pose sequences begin and is also a resting pose for all standing postures. If at any time you need a break when practicing standing poses, returning to this pose is the correct thing to do. As you see in the picture, the pose can be practiced with a chair to the front or side of you, this can help if you feel your balance is a bit off. Place your feet under your hips, either together, hip distance apart, or wider, then, ask yourself, where do I feel balanced and comfortable and put your feet there. Try to get your body weight evenly distributed through your feet and keep your feet parallel to each other. Your knees will stay soft in gentle yoga (some yoga styles do lock the knees), but the thigh muscles are active. You can gently tuck your tailbone, keep your chest wide open and relax your shoulders. Your chin may be tipped down a bit with your arms at your sides, or you can place your hands together in the center of your chest. If you are holding onto a chair, relax your arms and hands to keep from squeezing the chair. Your belly moves out as you inhale and your belly button pulls back toward your spine on the exhale. Keep your focal point on the floor right in front of you if you are a beginner, but when you want more challenge, move the focus farther away or close your eyes. In gentle yoga, we begin holding the posture for a breath or two, working up to five breaths and then when ready, hold it even longer.

Date _____

How did you do? Write out your comments about this pose.

_____

_____

Tall Mountain or Raised Hands Pose (Urdhva Hastasana)

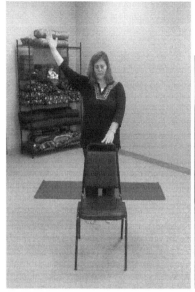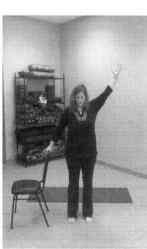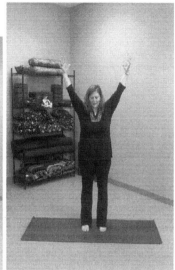

Tall Mountain pose is a standing pose with the arms stretched upwards. There are many ways to modify and adjust this pose to provide support and balance. You can place a chair in front of you, or to your side, for this pose. Begin in Mountain pose. Check your feet to make sure they are not splayed out as they should be parallel, and then slowly raise your hands over your head. Try to relax your shoulder blades down into your back pockets. Your arms can be out wide, straight up, or with your hands pressed together in the steeple position. Pick your favorite pose. Keep your hands down on the chair if you feel more comfortable that way. Your focal point can be on the floor right in front of you if you are a beginner, and if you want more challenge, move the focus farther away or close your eyes. This little movement challenges your balance.

In yoga we use a variety of breathing techniques while practicing the poses. You can adjust your breath to adjust other things going on around you. While breathing is usually automatic, you *can* control it. One example of control is holding your breath. One of the reasons yoga teachers are always talking about the breath is because it is so easy to hold your breath when concentrating on a pose and it's very important to keep breathing through the pose.

Date _____

How did you do? Write out your comments about this pose.

Crescent Moon or C-curve

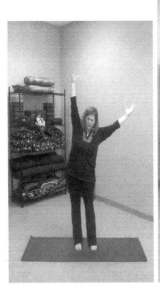 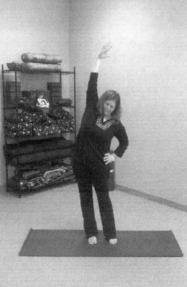 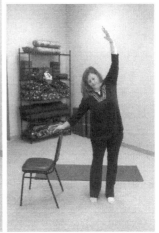

This is a simple side stretch. From the Tall Mountain pose, lean to one side creating a wide C with your body. Keep your abdominals firm to protect your lower back. You can also bring your feet out to a wider, more comfortable distance apart. If you have any back pain, avoid this pose or stay high, i.e. do not "C" too much, it should look more like a bent "I". Your hands can stay at your sides, or you can put your hands on your hip if it is too tiring to have your hands in the air. You also can hold on to the back of a chair or place one hand on the wall. There are many ways to modify and adjust this pose to provide support and balance. Keep your focal point on the floor right in front of you if you are a beginner, and if you want challenge, move the focus farther away or close your eyes.

A loud and energizing breathing technique, sometimes called the *HAH Breath*, can be done after this pose. Go back to Tall Mountain pose. Stand up tall, arms high, legs wide. Grab your hands together over your head and inhale. Drop your arms between your legs like you are chopping wood, and at the same time yell "Hah" loudly with the exhale. Inhale deeply again as you bring your hands back over your head. As you exhale, chop some wood and yell Hah again.

Date _____

How did you do? Write out your comments about this pose.

_____

_____

Five Pointed Star

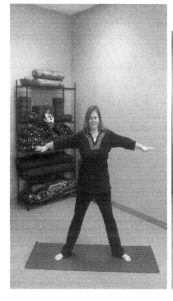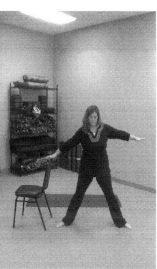

Five pointed star is a resting pose and a transition pose, a pose we often do to get from one pose to another. You can begin by placing your feet in a wide stance, 2- 3 feet apart with your toes facing out. Stretch your arms out and reach your fingertips out. Your arms will stay parallel to floor, although if your arms are tired, they may sag a bit. Reach the crown of your head to the ceiling and press your feet into the floor. Your shoulder blades will move a bit towards each other. Stretch your fingertips away from each other and imagine you can reach the opposite walls. This is an active pose, lengthening your arms and engaging your muscles. If your arms and shoulders get tired, place your hands on your hips or let them come down. Feel free to hold the wall, or a chair, for balance and rest. This pose can also be done sitting in a chair. The focal point can be in front of you, on the floor, or for more challenge, close your eyes.

In yoga, the breath is sometimes called prana. Prana is considered universal energy that balances the body and the mind. In science, this would equate to a balance between the sympathetic and the parasympathetic nervous systems. In yoga the breath is used to communicate between the body-mind systems, which gives us a tool to help facilitate positive change. For example, a deep belly breath brings the mind to the present moment and allows the body a fresh supply of nutrients.

Date _____

How did you do? Write out your comments about this pose.

Standing Spinal Twist (Sama Matsyendrasana)

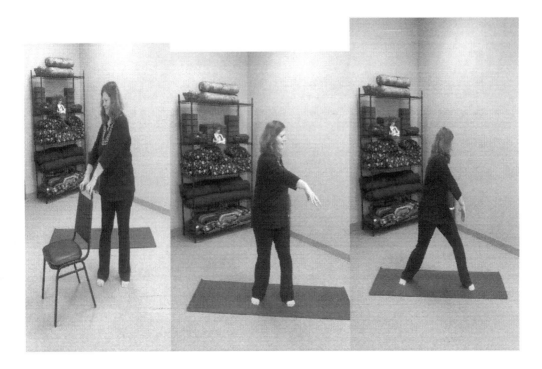

This is a standing twist often used in yoga warm-ups. It begins by planting your feet wider than your hips to stay balanced. You can initiate this pose from the five pointed star pose if you adjust your feet in a little. Stretch your arms out, parallel to the floor, then flop them from one side to the other while twisting at the waist. Swing side to side. Add a bit more swing if it feels good. You can also add a body slap, letting your arms and hands flop around. If you want to add a mini-twist, hold on each side for a breath or two. This is a great warm-up to loosen your arms and waist, but be careful to not twist too far or too fast. You can always hold a chair on each side if you need something to grab onto.

Breathing is the only bodily function we do both voluntarily and involuntarily. We can consciously use breathing to influence the involuntary system (sympathetic nervous system) which regulates blood pressure, heart rate, circulation, digestion and many other functions. So, as you do your poses, do not hold your breath.

Date _____

How did you do? Write out your comments about this pose.

Standing Forward Bend (Uttanasana)

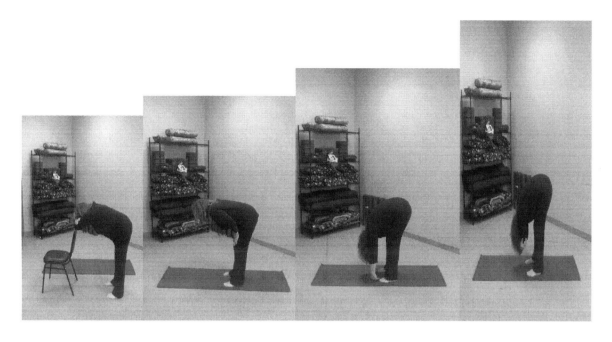

This is a basic forward bending pose with many variations. From Mountain pose, adjust your feet so they feel grounded and comfortable under you. Stand tall and reach your hands out wide in and a T position, with the fingertips reaching toward the walls. Fold your body from the hips, keeping your back flat, like you are folding a piece of paper. Stop half way and adjust to a flat back. Some people like to adjust their toes in a tiny bit to release their lower back. You can stay at halfway, rest with a chair, place your hands on your thighs, or continue to move your head lower toward your feet. You can have blocks waiting for you and allow your hands to drop to the blocks. Next, fold yourself at the hips, and imagine you have long hair which sweeps the floor and relax your neck. Deep forward bends like this can be a wonderful release for some people although problematic for others who experience problems with the low back, spinal discs, sciatica, or have neck injuries, high blood pressure, glaucoma, eye issues, headaches, or migraines. These reasons are why many people keep their head high and use a chair or rest their hands on their thighs. Keep your focal point at the floor at first, and then if you are very low, look back between your legs and feet.

Date _____

How did you do? Write out your comments about this pose.

_____

_____

Gentle Standing Back Bend (Anuvittasana)

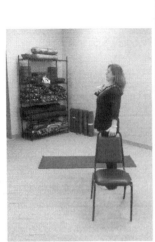 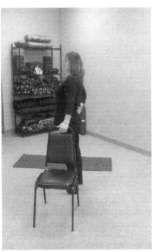 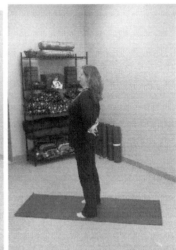

From Mountain, adjust your feet so they feel grounded and comfortable, as wide apart as you like. Place your hands on your low back if that feels safer. Lift your chest up and bend backwards a few inches. Keep your chin down or lift it to gaze at the place where the ceiling meets the wall. This is a mini-backbend and a slight chest opener. People with balance challenges may want to hold the chair or place a hand on the wall. Be extra careful or avoid backbends all together if you have disc or low back problems, sciatica, neck injuries, or chest tightness. If you have challenges with your neck, you can tuck your chin and look to the wall or the ground.

Are you a Chest Breather? Come back to the Mountain pose and place your right hand on your chest and your left hand on your abdomen. As you breathe, see which hand rises more. If your right hand rises more, you are a chest breather. If your left hand rises more, you are an abdomen breather. In yoga, we try to move away from breathing high in the chest, or what we call chest breathing. It is inefficient because the greatest amount of blood flow occurs in the lower lobes of the lungs. Rapid, shallow chest breathing high in the upper lungs results in less oxygen going into the blood. This results in less nutrients moving to the tissues. If you are under stress, your breathing may be high up in the lungs. If you are relaxed, breathing doesn't rely on the chest wall, but rather on the abdomen.

Date _____

How did you do? Write out your comments about this pose.

_____

_____

Gentle Chair (Utkatasana)

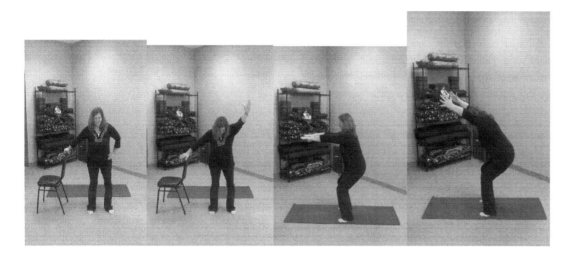

Begin in Mountain, and take a small step out to widen your stance. Decide if you want to have a chair next to you for support. As you bend your knees, keep your hips low. Move slowly and stop when you feel you need to. Next, think about where you want your hands. You can either keep them on your hips, bring your arms out in front of you, keep them at your sides, or up to frame your head. As you sink your hips towards floor, keep your back flat, and the weight will stay in your heels. Practice lifting up your toes and placing them down flat. Be careful if you have challenges with your knees or your balance. You can straighten the legs to take a rest, then do a forward fold and try again. You can also practice with your back flat against the wall or hold a strap to keep your arms in line. Try to keep your gaze forward.

Yoga includes ten timeless ethical principles, called the yamas and niyamas. These are positive guides for the yoga student's behavior. Some famous teachers have said there is no progress on the yogic path without these principles, meaning any prowess doing the physical postures is just calisthenics and ego unless the student is behaving in an ethical way too. This perspective makes the assumption that people can reform their behavior with positive thoughts, good habits, practice and repetition. This is what modern psychology has been concluding for years.

Date _____

How did you do? Write out your comments about this pose.

_____

_____

17

Gentle Wide Leg Forward Bend (Prasarita Padottanasana)

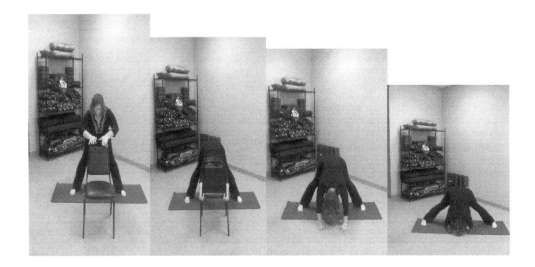

Decide if you want to have a chair in front of you for support while doing this deep forward bend, and if yes, place it a few feet in front of you. From the 5 pointed star pose, adjust your feet parallel, like skis. Stand tall and reach your hands out wide, so your fingertips are reaching to the walls, or, if you have a chair in front of you, hold both hands on the chair. Fold your body from the hips, like we did in Forward Fold, keeping your back flat. Stop halfway and adjust again to a flat back. Some people like to adjust their toes in a tiny bit. You can stay here and rest your hands on your hips or on the chair, and this is recommended for anyone with osteoporosis. If you want to move lower, continue bringing your hands to the floor. If your hands hit the floor, try to line your fingertips up with your toes, or place your elbows on the floor. Imagine you are completely releasing your neck. Do not put pressure on your head if it hits the ground. I always tell my students that you should be able to slip a piece of paper under your head. If you find it is too easy to reach to the top of the chair, flip it around and place your hands on the seat. You can also have blocks waiting for you so the hands will move to the blocks. The entire pose can be done sitting on a chair, too. Keep your focal point down toward the bottom of the wall or the floor. To come out of this pose can be challenging, so if needed put your hands on thighs, rise up slowly, move back to Mountain Pose and then try a gentle standing back bend.

Date _____

How did you do? Write out your comments about this pose.

Supported Pyramid or Intense Side Stretch (Parsvottanasana)

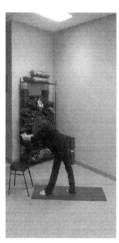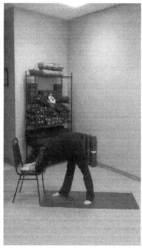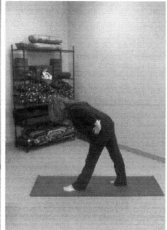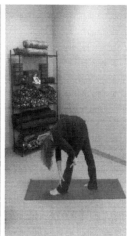

From Mountain, step one foot forward. Legs should stay straight but do not lock your knees. Place your hands on your hips. Fold your body from the hips, keeping your back flat. You can stay here and rest your hands on your hips or continue to move lower, bringing your hands to the floor, some blocks or a chair. If your hands hit the floor, one hand should be placed to each side of the front foot. Your arms can also wrap around your back and your chin can rest on your knee. Be extra careful if you have low blood pressure or are pregnant. You can place a chair in front of you and grab the chair top or seat if you like, or you can have blocks waiting for you so your hands can move to the blocks. Your eyes can rest on the wall, then move to the floor, one to two feet past your front foot. If you move lower, look at your shin. To come out of this pose can be challenging, so if needed walk your hands up your legs slowly, adjust yourself back to Mountain Pose and then try a gentle standing back bend.

Come back to Mountain Pose to practice Abdominal Breathing (also called Diaphragmatic Breathing). The diaphragm is a large muscle located between the chest and the abdomen. By expanding the lung's air pockets and improving the flow of blood and lymph, abdominal breathing helps prevent infections in the lungs. This type of breathing will also help stimulate your relaxation response. Abdominal breathing allows control of your breath and will help you focus on the moment. Put your hands on your abdomen, with three fingers below your navel. As you breathe in, your abdomen should rise, like a balloon inflating. As you breathe out your abdomen should fall like a balloon losing air.

Date _____

How did you do? Write out your comments about this pose.

_____

_____

Gentle Triangle (Utthita Trikonasana)

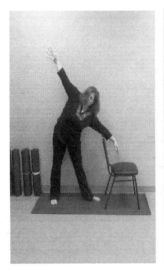 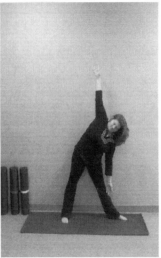

From 5 Pointed Star, adjust both feet toward one wall. One foot should turn parallel to the mat and the other will be on an angle. Keep your arms out to your side and parallel to the floor. Imagine the finger over the foot parallel to the mat is being hooked and pulled over that foot, like you are being pulled from the waist. When you have reached your "edge" and stop naturally, windmill your arms. One arm now stretches up toward the ceiling and the other reaches for the floor. This lower hand can find support on your shin, thigh, a chair or the floor. Be careful if you have low blood pressure, neck injuries, or any back problems. If you want to adjust this pose, bend your knee and keep your lower hand on the inside of your thigh or shin. Your eyes can look at the floor, wall or ceiling. To come out of the pose move to 5 Pointed Star and set your feet up to do the pose on the other side. A good after stretch is the Standing Forward Bend.

Move back to the Mountain Pose to begin some abdominal breathing. As you inhale, try to make a light snore sound in the back of your throat. The breath is not forced, but regular and peaceful. This is called Ocean Sounding Breath or Ujjayi Breath. When practicing this breath, teachers will introduce breathing rhythms like Savitri Pranayama which is a 2-1-2-1 breath. Inhale to the count of 2, hold for the count of 1, exhale to the count of 2 and pause for the count of 1. There are many other rhythms suggested by teachers, but in Gentle Yoga it most important to be aware of your breath and especially not to hold your breath.

Date _____

How did you do? Write out your comments about this pose.

_____

_____

_____

Gentle Revolved Triangle (Parivrtta Trikonasana)

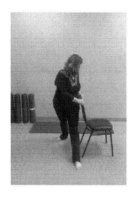 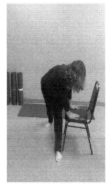 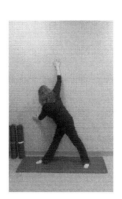

This pose can be difficult for many people, including me, so this is a Gentle Yoga variation I enjoy. With your feet set up like in the Triangle Pose and your back to the wall, place your hands on your hips. Twist and face the wall adjusting your feet for comfort. Reach out to the wall and position your hands, one high and one low, leaning on the wall. Press your chest and shoulders flat against the wall, if possible. Then begin to inch your bottom fingers down the wall and try to inch raised fingers up the wall. (If you feel flexible, sweep your arms around like a windmill and see where they land). Use common sense and be careful if you have migraines, low blood pressure, rotator cuff issues, spine or neck injuries as this may not be the pose for you. To modify this pose further, stay high on the wall and work on breathing evenly in this gentle twist. You may not get flat against the wall, a tight waist or tight shoulders may stop you, but this is the place to begin. If you like, let your lower hand fall to the ground near your foot and reach your high hand to the sky. Keep your eyes focused in front of you and, if you are comfortable, look up. Do not twist or crank your neck or low back. Slowly come out of the pose and if you want a counter stretch try the Standing Forward Bend.

As I mentioned, I find this pose more challenging now than I did years ago. Because of this, it is a perfect time to practice one of the ethical principles of yoga, non-violence, and its positive ideal, compassion. Twisting and cranking my neck or low back would demonstrate a complete lack of compassion for myself at this stage of life. Compassion for yourself is front and center in gentle yoga, especially when we encounter frustration, as I do in this pose. As you move through the poses in this book, please be kind to yourself and remember to apply the principle of non-violence.

Date _____

How did you do? Write out your comments about this pose.

21

Crescent Lunge (Alanasana is sometimes used)

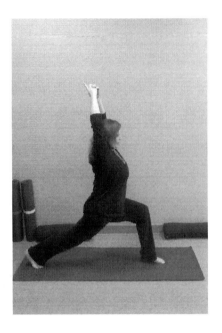

Crescent Lunge is a powerful pose similar to the Warrior 1 pose, but the back heel is lifted and you press into the ball of your foot instead of dropping your foot to the mat at an angle. I always say the arm placement is variable. Teachers will guide this pose in different ways, for example, putting the hands together at heart center or the arms up to steeple position. To begin, your front knee is bent and you should be able to see your big toe. Balancing can be a challenge so adjust your stance a few times to see where the right position is for you. You can hold the wall or a chair if this helps. Your focus should be a few feet in front of your toe on the floor or straight ahead. Your shoulders relax and the crown of your head reaches towards the sky.

When you have practiced a few lunges, try *Ujjayi Cleansing Breath.* This is the deep Ocean Sounding breath, but just like the Mommy Breath it is a reset breath and can include a big sigh. Inhale and exhale quickly using the light snore sound in the back of the throat. You may want to add a loud sigh and make it fun.

Date _____

How did you do? Write out your comments about this pose.

_____

_____

Low Lunge (Anjaneyasana)

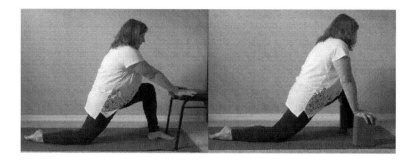

Low Lunge is similar to the Crescent Lunge, but in this pose your back lower leg will have the knee and shin resting on the floor (or a little higher if needed). The placement of your arms is variable, and your hands can be at heart center or resting on a chair. Your front knee is bent and you should be able to see your big toe. Balancing can be a challenge for many people, especially as we get older. You can adjust your stance a few times to see where your body is comfortable. You can hold the wall or a chair if this helps. There are many ways to modify and adjust this pose to provide comfort, support and balance. Your eyes should focus at the floor a few feet in front of the toe or straight ahead if you feel balanced in the pose. Relax your shoulders and allow the crown of your head to reach toward the sky.

You have probably heard about yogis eating a vegan diet and not wearing animal fur. They do this out of compassion for animals and the hungry and out of respect for the planet. But this principle goes far beyond avoiding meat in your diet. It includes the elimination of violence in all forms: war, crime, fictional violence, and even violence toward yourself. The advanced practice is the elimination of thoughts and even dreams of violence. It seems strange and impossible to imagine an entire world like this, free from all thought and acts of violence, but this is the mindset of the yogi. In these poses continue to practice compassion for yourself.

Date _____

How did you do? Write out your comments about this pose.

23

Small Stance Warrior I (Virabhadrasana I)

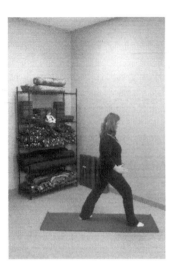 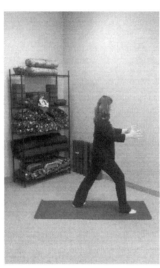 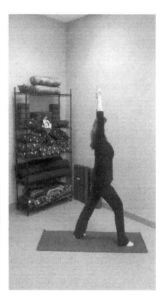

From Mountain, put your hands on your hips and step back with your right foot. Squaring your hips to the front wall, bend your front leg and adjust your stance so you feel balanced. When you feel grounded and balanced, sweep your arms up and decide if you are most comfortable with your arms parallel to each other, in a "V", or in steeple position (or if you like keep the hands on your hips). In any pose like this you can tighten and release your core muscles to protect your back. If you feel balanced, close your eyes, otherwise keep your gaze on one focal point on the floor and breathe.

Date _____

How did you do? Write out your comments about this pose.

_____

_____

Warrior II (Virabhadrasana II)

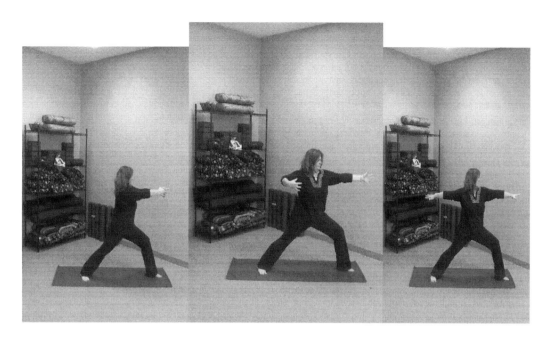

From Warrior 1, drop your hands in front of you and reach toward the front. Then, pretend you are pulling a bow back so one hand will move behind you. When you have pulled all the way back, flip the palms of each hand down. Glance over your front outstretched arm. Check that your front knee is bent but that you can still see your toes. You should feel strong and grounded. Think about the future in front of you, the past behind you and be steady and grounded in the present moment. When we talk about the present moment we are not obliterating the past or the future, or pretending they do not exist, we are just staying firm in the present. Your hands may rest on your hips, and your front leg can be straightened at any time if you get tired. You can hold a chair or the wall for balance. Glance over the fingertips of your outstretched arm and keep your gaze focused and steady.

Date _____

How did you do? Write out your comments about this pose.

Reverse Warrior (Viparita Virabhadrasana)

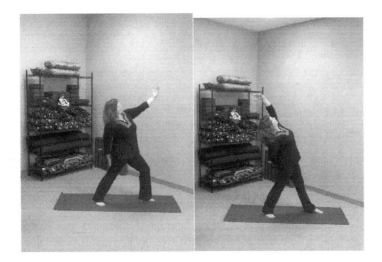

From Warrior II, flip your front palm and raise it up to the sky. As you sweep this arm to the sky, lower your back arm to rest on your thigh. A slight backbend will occur naturally, but beware of going too deep. To make the pose more gentle do not look up, keep your front arm low or do not put too much arch in your back. Also you can hold a chair or the wall instead of resting that back hand on the back leg. Your focal point will be the fingertips of the overhead arm. To counter the pose you can do any forward bend.

In the 1800s one of the fathers of American psychology, William James, thought our character was as solid as a rock by the age of 30. Modern psychologists would agree, that while there are certain personality traits that seem fixed (like introversion and extroversion), we now know the brain is plastic and continues to learn throughout life. Events and environments can alter an individual's behavior. With practice we approach the yogic system as a developmental process with new learning building on itself.

Date _____

How did you do? Write out your comments about this pose.

_____

_____

Gentle Extended Side Angle (Utthita Parsvakonasana)

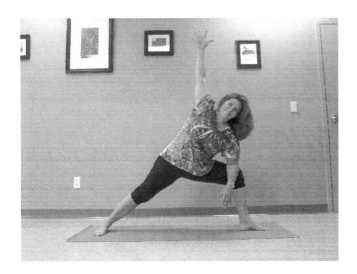

Here I am pictured in one of my old studio spaces. I miss that old place! From Warrior II, bring the elbow above the bent knee and down to rest on the knee. Feel free to drop this hand to a block or the floor, or even behind the foot on the floor, if placement on the knee is too easy for you. Continue to reach your outstretched arm to the ceiling or begin to stretch it over your ear to make a straight line from fingers to foot. Some people say this can relieve mild sciatica, but if you have sciatica, be careful. I know that it shows up differently in each individual. The pose will feel like it lengthens your spine. Be careful with this pose if you have low blood pressure or knee injuries. If it bothers you to put your elbow on your knee, just rest your hand there. If you have trouble with balance, lean against a wall, hold on to chair, or use a smaller stance. When you feel a comfort level in the pose, find a focal point a few feet away.

Date _____

How did you do? Write out your comments about this pose.

_____

_____

Gentle Balance Poses

Imagine this familiar scenario playing out in your life. Late in the afternoon, around 5 p.m., a bewitching hour. You are standing at the stove trying to whip-up a meal for your family. You are exhausted from a long day, and a hungry preschooler who wants attention is underfoot. Your school-aged child is yelling about needing a new spiral notebook for fourth period tomorrow, and you envision a late night trip to the superstore. Your husband walks in, regal and majestic after a long day in the cube, sniffing around for his food like a dog looking for a tender bone. Your breath becomes short, quick, high in the chest. What do you do as the stress mounts? Then, you remember, yogic breathing. As you take deep belly breaths, slow and easy, over and over, you calmly complete the dish on the stove, lift the preschooler for a kiss, and out of the corner of your eye see an extra spiral notebook on your desk that will work quite nicely. Seriously though, yogic breathing can help greatly reduce anxiety.

Yogic breathing helps with balance as well. Pranayama is the fourth limb of yoga out of 8 limbs. It literally means the control of life or energy. This refers to the breathing techniques yogis use to change subtle energies within the body for good health. Breathing acts as a bridge to deeper meditation in yoga.

In addition to calm breath, finding a focal point will be very helpful for balance. I often tell my students to look for a bit of dust or a spot on the floor to use for a focal point. I have also taken out shiny objects or shells and placed them on the floor to use as a focal point. Some people will prefer a spot on the opposite wall. It really is more important that you find a focal point then what it looks like. As you practice these balance poses first make sure you are safe and can hold onto something if needed. Then breathe rhythmically and do not hold the breath. Finally, find a good focal point and keep your eyes on it. When you feel more confident you can always close your eyes.

Half Moon (Ardha Chandrasana)

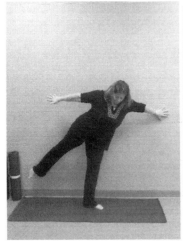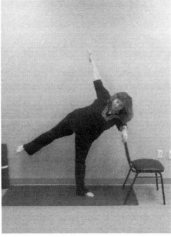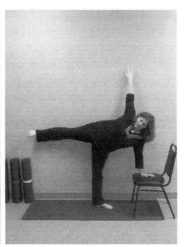

One of the gods, Ganesh, was mad at the moon and threw a tusk at it, darkening the sky. Eventually he let the moon shine again but it was forced to wax and wane. The pose represents dark and light and the value of opposites. We would not want every day to be the same.

For this pose, you may want to begin flat against a wall with a chair next to you. Begin in Mountain. Practice lifting one foot a few inches to the side and reaching your opposite arm out (maybe reaching to a chair). Hold the top of the chair or the seat of the chair, depending on what is most comfortable for you to begin with. Slowly work to lift the outstretched leg a bit more while your hand rests on the top of a chair or the seat of a chair. If your back leans on the wall for support, pretend the wall is not really there. This is a pose you may want to avoid if you have problems with balance, your back, sciatica, neck injuries, knees, or vertigo.

You also can get on your knees and do this pose against the wall. Feel free to use a chair, the wall or blocks. You can focus on the ceiling, the wall or look down; whatever helps you to balance. Don't forget to do the pose on both sides. You can counter this pose with standing forward bend.

Date _____

How did you do? Write out your comments about this pose.

_____

_____

Warrior III (Virabhadrasana III)

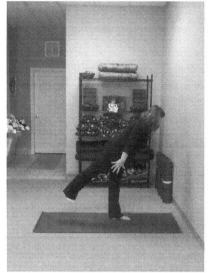 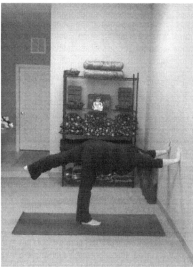 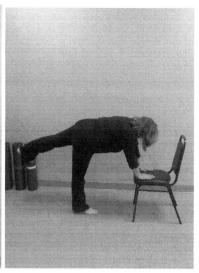

From Mountain pose facing a wall, put your arms down and stand like a soldier. Lift one foot a tiny bit off the floor and lean a bit forward. Move your arms out in front of you, reaching to the wall. Place your hands or elbows flat on the wall for support. Start your hands high on the wall and then experiment with moving them down the wall. You can also experiment with continuing to lift the one raised leg. Try a little farther from the wall. Work toward a flat back, allowing the whole body to form a "T". Breathe. This pose can really challenge your balance, which is why we stand near the wall. You can also reach to a chair, but make sure it is a heavy one which will not tip over. This pose is also good for stretching your hips. Be careful if you have any trouble with your ankles, feet or knees. Keep your focus steady by looking at a spot down on the floor.

Date _____

How did you do? Write out your comments about this pose.

_____

_____

Tree (Vrksasana)

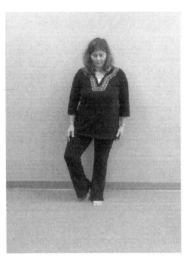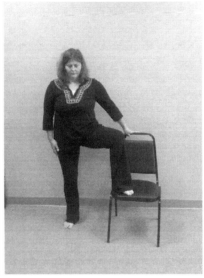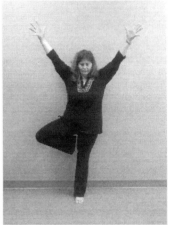

There are many ways to modify and adjust Tree pose to provide support and balance, and I find many students prefer to use a chair or wall when practicing this pose. From Mountain pose, shift your weight onto your left foot. Then, bend your right knee and bring it out to side, finding a comfortable place to rest the sole of your foot along the inside leg, avoiding the knee joint (ankle, calf or thigh area is fine). Your toes can stay on floor for balance if that is more comfortable, and the arms can stay down. You can place your hands on your hips, out to sides, high in the air, or in front of your chest. This pose can help with balance but you do not want to fall, so holding a chair or the wall for safety is recommended at first. In all balancing poses the focal point is critical. It can be a foot or two in front of your foot to begin with. Rest in the Mountain pose when you come out of this standing balance pose, holding the chair or wall if you like.

One of the ethical principles in yoga is honesty. It begins with speaking the truth, but does not stop there. It encompasses other behaviors such as insincerity, compulsive lying, faking your emotions, denial and procrastination. This is an interesting time in history to promote this principle because according to recent research narcissism is on the rise. Serious, and culture altering, dishonesty happens in politics, government corruption or taxpayer bailouts.

Date _____

How did you do? Write out your comments about this pose.

_____

_____

Dancer (King Dancer Pose – Natarajasana)

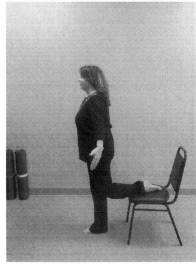 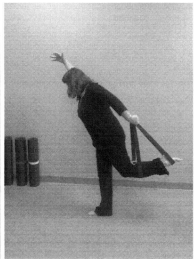 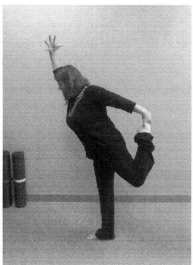

There are many ways to modify and adjust this pose to provide support and balance. Begin by shifting your weight onto your left foot. Inhale while moving your right arm up in the air and just slightly lift the right foot. If it is hard to balance, place the left hand on a chair or use the wall. Lift the right foot up towards your buttocks and attempt to grab your ankle. If it is impossible to reach your ankle or holding the foot is uncomfortable, just keep your leg elevated and imagine you are holding your foot. If you do reach your ankle, press your foot into that hand while inhaling. If you feel balanced or have a good grip on the chair, hinge forward and allow the foot you are holding to move towards ceiling. Often, the hardest part is keeping your hips square to floor. This can challenge even the best balancers, so feel free to grip the wall or chair at all times, and avoid this pose if you have shoulder or lower back issues. You can also use a strap to hold your foot, but this can make the pose even more difficult if the strap gets in your way. Your focal point will depend on where you are in the pose, either a few feet in front of you or looking up to the ceiling.

This is one of the most popular images of yoga on the internet. You can search this picture and see some amazing yoga images but the pose can be done with full support and using props with similar results.

Date _____

How did you do? Write out your comments about this pose.

_____

_____

Hand to Big Toe (Utthita Hasta Padangusthasana)

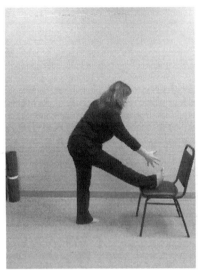 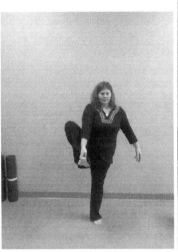 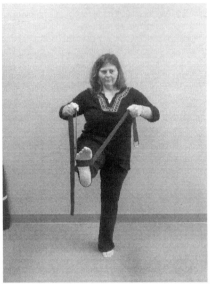

This is another balancing pose where you may find the wall or chair a wonderful prop. From Mountain, shift your weight onto your left foot. Bend your right knee and hold it in front of you. Slowly reach down and grab your toe. You may need to hold it here for a minute. Begin to stretch the leg out in front. If you need a little help reaching your toes you can grab the foot with a strap and hold the whole leg up with it. If you want to experiment with balance, slowly swing your leg out to the side (with or without the strap). Find a focal point in front of you. Hold, breathe, and move back to Mountain pose before trying this on the other side.

The combination of the first two ethical principles of yoga, truth telling and nonviolence, should be practiced together but can be tricky. When telling the truth is violent and hurtful to another, we are breaking the first yama. Think of all the people who begin conversations with, "I don't mean to criticize you but..." and go on a rant that is critical. Even if every criticism cited has a basis in reality, the verbal violence is unmistakable and unnecessary. Practicing satya means we yield to compassion and keep our mouth shut. To practice satya, yoga teachers advise us to let go of voicing strong opinions and to speak carefully and deliberately. There are very few people who model of this type of careful and deliberate speech, maybe because it is not rewarded in our culture, but if you do find a teacher like this you have found gold.

Date _____

How did you do? Write out your comments about this pose.

_____

_____

Eagle Pose (Garudasana)

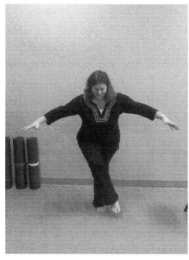 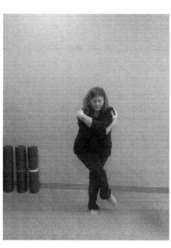 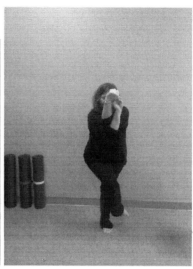

From Mountain, shift your weight onto your left foot. Lift your right knee, bring your whole leg around the front of your other leg, balancing on your left leg. Your left knee will be bent. You can leave the leg resting over the other, or curl the right leg around the left. This will strengthen core muscles and help you balance. Feel free to hold a wall or a chair to help. When you feel strong on your legs, and if your arms are free, give yourself a little hug. Find a focal point a bit past your knee or on the wall in front of your foot. Return to Mountain pose before trying this on the other side.

There is no doubt an eagle is a bird of prey, but it does not take more prey than it needs. A plant does not take more sun and water than it requires. But humans accumulate and build and hoard. A basic principle in yoga is do not steal. It is more than just resisting the urge to grab a candy bar from the rack near the cash register, it includes avoiding taking or buying things which you do not need. Some advanced yogis would call stealing mental illness, and clinical psychologists that work with hoarders would agree. It takes extreme discipline to not want things, the wider culture will always try to tell you what you need, what to buy, how to live. Advertising and new products are everywhere. Most people find balance but for some it is impossible to resist acquiring things.

Date _____

How did you do? Write out your comments about this pose.

Gentle Prone Poses

The set of poses presented here are prone poses, meaning you are face down in a surrender position. For those who practice yoga for spiritual reasons the prone poses will always bring the thoughts to devotion, sacrifice, surrender and letting go of selfishness. Some of the poses take a lot of strength and discipline, but at the same time there is a sense of humility.

The first thing to do is think of a way to move to the floor that is safe for you. Each person is different and some people will use the chair or a wall to move from standing to the floor. If you can get down on the floor comfortably, stay there and select a few of these poses you find comfort in. You may need props for some of these poses. Try not to view the props as a crutch or weakness, they are available to help you, and will make your poses stronger. You can gain the same exact benefits of yoga if you use props, a calm mind and peaceful spirit. Please don't avoid props if they make you more comfortable.

Table Pose (Utpithikasana)

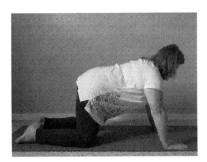

Like many yogis, I do not know the history or origins of the Table Pose. Table pose is often used as a resting pose, or part of the Cat-Cow spinal warm up series of poses outlined below. Many people hate to be on their knees or wrists like this so I always suggest a blanket under the knees if needed, coming down to the forearms if needed, or getting out of the pose all together if it is really uncomfortable. That said, if you are coming to the mat from a standing position, carefully work yourself down to your hands and knees and use a chair to lower yourself to the floor. Place your hands under your shoulders with straight arms. Your back will be flat, in one straight line, like a table top. Your knees will be under the hips, and your shins and the tops of your feet will rest on the floor.

Bramacharya, or managing your personal energy, gets a lot of attention in yogic circles because at one time some popular gurus encouraged celibacy for yoga students. But, this moral restraint actually addresses all forms of addiction. Addictions can be harmful and can often hurt people close to us, which is why this is a social discipline. Addiction is also antisocial, a waste of personal talent and when in its grip, you withhold from the world the gifts you have been blessed with. For this reason yogis curb addictions.

Date _____

How did you do? Write out your comments about this pose.

_____

_____

Cat (Marjaryasana)

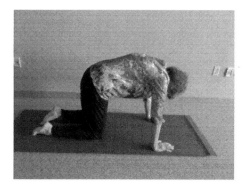

From Table Pose arch your back to the sky like an angry cat. Round the entire spine, including the neck, so the crown of the head is now facing downward. You can stay in the pose for a few breaths or come back to Table Pose to rest. If you enjoy the cat pose, stay in it for a while.

Generosity is considered an advanced yoga practice because it is so difficult for some to give freely, without the expectation of a return. Sharing from a place of abundance lifts everyone up. The final yama, aparigraha, or non-possessiveness, is letting go of greed and giving generously to others, be it money or time or help.

Date _____

How did you do? Write out your comments about this pose.

Cow (Bitilasana)

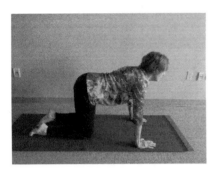

The Cow Pose usually follows the Cat Pose or Table Pose. From either of these poses, drop your belly towards the ground so your back is arching the opposite of the Cat Pose in a deep U. Your low spine is higher than the mid-spine. your shoulders are strong and now the crown of your head is tilting upwards.

The personal disciplines, known in yoga as niyamas, are very practical and contribute to transformation no matter your age. The first personal discipline, purity, refers to cleanliness of body, home, and other surroundings you may find yourself in. It includes juice cleansing, but also letting go of what is unnecessary and becoming free from material attachments. It may be hard to determine what to get rid of, but a yoga practice will help hone your ability to do this more easily.

Date _____

How did you do? Write out your comments about this pose.

Spinal Balance

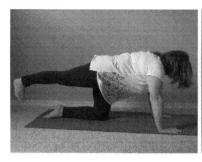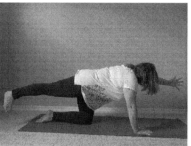

Spinal Balancing can be practiced after Cat and Cow. Begin in Table Pose, lift your right leg and stretch it away from your body. Point and flex your toes. Reach it out and straighten your leg so it is parallel to the floor. Return to Table Pose, rest, and lift your left leg, holding it about the same amount of time as the first leg. Go back to Table Pose, rest, and lift your right arm, stretch it out, wiggle your fingers, breathe and place it back down. Then lift your left arm. To challenge yourself, lift your left leg and right arm at the same time. Then your right leg along with your left arm.

Balancing poses are a staple in yoga. These poses teach us about contentment, or santosha, challenging us to see beyond our material goals and to be satisfied with what we have now. It does not mean we tolerate substandard things, but the practice encourages us to focus on gratitude in the moment and not the unknown future. For some people satisfaction is not enough, they have to be happy. Replacing contentment with amped-up happiness leads people to feeling unfulfilled if that happiness eludes them. Studies find you can increase your happiness by practicing gratitude, which is another way of saying be content with what you have.

Date _____

How did you do? Write out your comments about this pose.

41

Classic Child's Pose (Balasana)

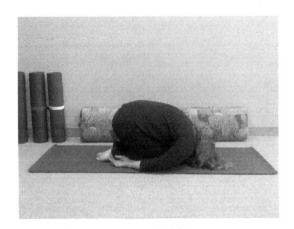

Child's Pose is a resting pose, a counter pose for many postures and a crowd favorite. From kneeling, lean forward, sit back on your heels and rest your chest on your thighs. The weight of your head rests on your forehead. Wrap your arms around your body towards your feet for a classic pose or extend your arms out for the Extended Child pose. Your knees can also be wide, resting your torso in-between your thighs. You can rest your forehead or chest on bolsters for a Restorative Child's Pose. Close eyes.

Date _____

How did you do? Write out your comments about this pose.

_____

_____

Runner's Lunge (Alanasana is sometimes used)

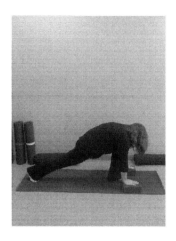

Runner's Lunge is similar to the other lunges described, Crescent Lunge and Low Lunge, but now your hands or forearms stay on the ground and your face is positioned down, making it more of a surrender pose as opposed to a strength pose. Your arm placement is straight under your shoulders and blocks can be used if it is hard to fit your leg or knee below the chest. Your front knee is bent. Your back foot is pressing into the ball of the foot and your heel is up. Your eyes can focus between your hands. Shoulders should be relaxed.

Alana means rope or binding, so some yogis may have called this pose this name as a representation of being bound to the god Shiva or being a minister of Shiva. (As I have said before, yogis get creative.) Shiva was a god of yoga and action. The way yogis change the world is through action (like Gandhi). Karma yoga is another path of yoga where action, mind, body and spirit are all combined in a unique way. This yoga path is a disciplined practice designed to make it easier to persevere in the face of obstacles.

Date _____

How did you do? Write out your comments about this pose.

_____

_____

Plank (Kumbhakasana)

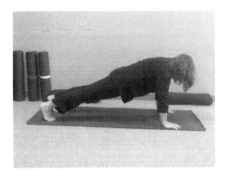

Plank Pose is a classic yoga pose, done in almost all yoga classes and known for strengthening the core, abdomen, chest, and lower back. It also strengthens the arms, wrists, spine muscles and shoulders. But, this pose can be very difficult for people in gentle yoga classes if the student has trouble with their wrists or shoulders. Plus, it can be very difficult to hold up your body weight for a long time so start slowly. You know you are making progress when you can hold this pose longer and longer each day.

From the table pose, make sure your wrists are directly under your shoulders. Spread your fingers and press down through your forearms and hands. Slowly, step back with your feet, one at a time, bringing your body and head into one straight line. Don't let your bottom get too high or too low. People with wrist and shoulder problems or carpel tunnel usually avoid this pose. If you drop your knees to the floor, it makes the pose much easier. This is called Half Plank which is the next pose described. Your focal point should be down. If you need to counter this pose with another pose, try child's pose.

Discipline and transformation (tapas) is important to yogis. But this does not come naturally. It is a practice of balancing austerity and sacrifice. In our culture, rigid dieting and exercise programs come to mind, but disciple includes keeping commitments, staying focused, honoring promises to others, and trying to avoid letting people down and disappointing them. Holding the plank position will require discipline.

Date _____

How did you do? Write out your comments about this pose.

_____

_____

Half Plank (Ardha Kumbhakasana)

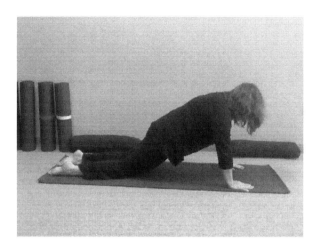

Half Plank Pose tones the core, abdomen, chest, and lower back. It strengthens the arms, wrists, spine muscles and shoulders. From the table pose, make sure your wrists are directly under your shoulders. Spread your fingers and press down through your forearms and hands. Slowly step back with your feet, one at a time, and drop your knees down. Your body and head will be in one straight line. Don't let your bottom get too high or too low. People with wrist and shoulder problems or carpel tunnel usually avoid this pose. Your hands can go on a folded blanket to ease your wrists, or roll mat a few times, place it under your wrists, and curl your fingers over the rolled mat. Your focal point should be down. If you need to counter this pose with another, try child's pose.

Plank and Half Plank are very challenging for some people, and they both enhance determination. When we are fired up about something, we need to balance determination and failure. Seeking out mentors who live a balanced life is important for anyone charting a new course. Self-study, getting to know yourself, trying not to judge yourself and attempting to inspire others are all parts of the yoga practice that assist us in balancing passionate determination with failure.

Date _____

How did you do? Write out your comments about this pose.

_____

_____

Dolphin Plank (Makara Adho Mukha Svanasana)

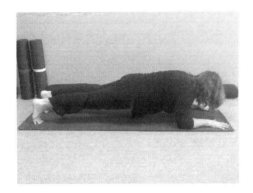

There are a few ways to begin this pose, some begin in plank or down dog, but I think it is easier to move to this pose from Table pose. Lower your forearms to the floor with your palms facing down. Adjust your elbows under your shoulders. Spread your fingers wide and press your hands into the mat. If you were in Table pose, place one leg back and then the other. Adjust your body so it is in one straight line, with your heels over your toes. Squeeze your abdominals tight. This makes even breathing a little harder but keep squeezing. Try to relax your lower muscles and the shoulders. Breathe. This pose is great for building your core, abdominal, and lower back muscles. Anyone with a shoulder injury or recent shoulder surgery will want to avoid this pose. You can always drop your knees down to make it easier (see next page). Some people place a folded blanket under their knees. Your focal point should be down or eyes closed. Move to Child's Pose to counter this pose if you like.

Dolphins are incredibly efficient, maybe because of the awesome way they communicate. As in the animal kingdom, waste is abhorred in yoga. In the US, 133 billion pounds of the available food supply went to waste in 2010. In yoga, this is considered stealing. When you think about the freshwater, land and energy used to get this food to consumers, an astonishing amount of waste is left in its wake if food is eventually tossed in the garbage. Some food is spoiled or rotten, some thrown away by retailers because it is blemished, some is just scraped off our plates into the trash can. If you do not buy what you cannot eat, you have saved time, money and national resources.

Date _____

How did you do? Write out your comments about this pose.

Half Dolphin Plank (Makara Adho Mukha Savasana)

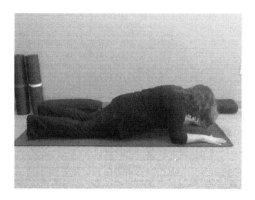

There are a few ways to begin this pose, but it is easiest to move from Table pose. Lower your forearms to the floor with your palms facing down. Adjust your elbows under your shoulders. Spread your fingers wide and press your hands into the mat. Place one leg back with knee down and then the other leg back with your knee down. Adjust your body so it is in one straight line. Your heels may be over your toes, or just rest your feet. Engage your abs here, pushing your belly button toward your spine on each exhale. Relax your gluteus, relax your shoulders. Breathe. This pose is good for your core, abs, and lower back muscles. Anyone with shoulder injury or recent upper body surgery may want to avoid this. Some people may like a folded blanket under their knees or elbows. Your focal point should be down or your eyes closed. Move to Child's Pose to counter this pose if you like.

In cultures of materialism and selfishness, surrender is not always valued or even discussed. It is viewed as weak. Yogis have a personal practice of surrender (also called ishvara-pranidhana) which can be found in a prayer or in a simple gesture of kindness which serves others. It can be surrender to a higher power or surrender to something other than our own agenda, plans or goals. This is letting go, not the letting go of an old pair of jeans, but letting go of control.

Date _____

How did you do? Write out your comments about this pose.

_____

_____

Down Dog (Adho Mukha Svanasana)

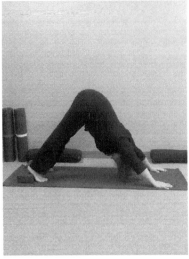 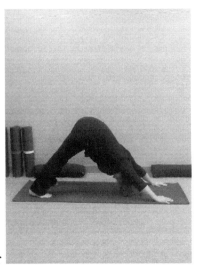

or

Downward facing dog is a transitional pose, a resting pose and a great strengthener in its own right. Sometimes it is done many times during a yoga class. From the Plank pose, lift your hips high in the air and back a little, drop your head between your straightened arms, and place your heels on the floor. If your hamstrings are tight, keep your heels up, maybe placing them on blocks. Some people just love Down Dog and rest in this pose. Some people find it much too hard on their wrists and shoulders. Although you may hear it called a resting pose, it can be very difficult for many people. This is why we bring in a chair as a prop. The focal point will naturally be down at the floor. If you need to counter this pose with another, try any gentle backbend.

At the end of the Mahabharata, an epic Indian poem, there is a story of a loyal and faithful dog, which is where the name of this pose may come from. In many other ancient myths (from all over the globe) dogs are not only guardians, hunting companions and best friends, but spiritual guides.

Date _____

How did you do? Write out your comments about this pose.

_____

_____

Down Dog (Adho Mukha Svanasana) with a chair as prop

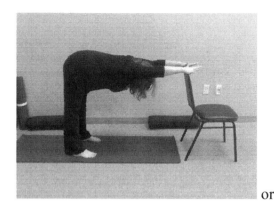 or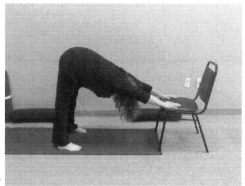

Although you may hear Downward Facing Dog referred to as a resting pose, it can be very difficult for many people without some help or support. This is why we bring in a chair as a prop. With the back of the chair in front of you, do a forward bend with a flat back, stretching your hands out to meet the chair. If you would like a little more challenge and you are comfortable with your head lower than your heart, flip the chair around and reach out for the seat. Try to keep your shoulders relaxed and your head between your arms. It is natural to keep your heels firmly on the ground while using a chair in this pose. Your focal point is naturally down at the floor. If you need to counter this pose with another, try any gentle standing backbend.

Many of my students resist using a prop (like a chair) at first. I feel like I have to sell them on the idea. Then, when they try it, they are in bliss. One great thing about yoga is that it challenges us to see beyond our material goals and our egos. It teaches us to be satisfied with what we have now, even if it is a body that needs a little support in a pose. We move to remedy a bad situation when needed but we are encouraged to focus on our gratitude for each moment and not dwell on the unknown future.

Date _____

How did you do? Write out your comments about this pose.

49

Upward Facing Dog (Urdhva Mukha Svanasana)

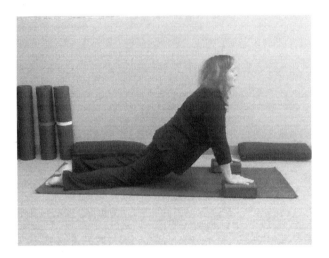

This is often used as a transitional pose in Sun Salutation, but can also be practiced alone. If this pose is too difficult, stay in Cobra or Sphinx. Or from Cobra, continue to push up and lift your thighs off the floor. Press the tops of your feet into floor. Lift your hips. The shoulders stay over your wrists, relaxed. This pose can strengthen your arms, wrists, and ankles. Watch out if you have wrist or shoulder problems, carpel tunnel syndrome, low back issues, pregnancy, serious back injury or disk problems. Drop into Sphinx arms if you need to take pressure off your wrists. Your thighs are down and your hips sink down. Your focal point should be one or two feet in front of your nose or, if you like, close your eyes to meditate. As you come out, stretch into Child's Pose.

Date _____

How did you do? Write out your comments about this pose.

Cobra (Bujangasana)

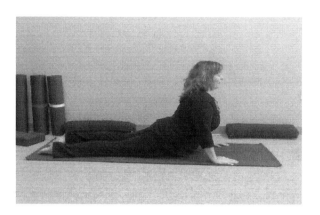

Lie face down, with your chin on the floor, hands next to shoulders. Press your pelvic triangle down. Stage 1-use your back muscles to lift your shoulders off the floor. Stage 2-Lift your chest off of the floor. Stage 3- lift your belly button off of the floor. Relax your shoulders down, elbows tucked into your ribs, your back is strong, gluteus soft, and your chest lifts. Your chin can be tucked or parallel to the floor. This pose strengthens the back muscles. If you have back or neck trouble, wrist problems, carpel tunnel or shoulder problems, you may not like this pose. In this case, do the pose in stages and stop at Stage 1 or 2, or do the Sphinx Pose listed below. Do not crank your head too far back and always protect your neck. You can use a folded blanket under your hands or hips if needed. Your focal point should be one or two feet in front of your nose or, if you like, close your eyes to meditate. As you come out, stretch into Child's Pose.

This pose may have been named after the cobra because the god Shiva has snakes draped around his neck and his son Ganesh has one tied around his waist. The cobra (or snake) represents death and fear. Yoga teaches us to try to master our fears. Fears need to be acknowledged and recognized and then they can be dealt with.

Date _____

How did you do? Write out your comments about this pose.

_____

_____

Sphinx (Salamba Bhujangasana)

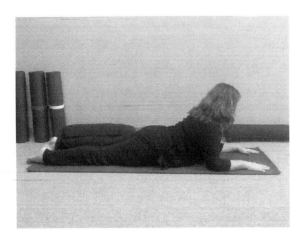

Sphinx opens the chest and strengthens the core body. Begin prone, with your forearms flat on the floor, elbows under your shoulders, legs together, and the top of your feet pressed to the floor. Press your forearms and hands down into the floor. Pull up your knee caps, squeeze your thighs and buttocks, and press your pubic bone down into the floor. Keep your elbows close to your sides. Press your chest forward. Keep your head neutral, with your chin parallel to the floor. Breathe. Avoid the pose if you have had recent or chronic injury to the back, arms or shoulders, are pregnant or recent abdominal surgery. You can use a folded blanket under your forearms. Your focal point should be one or two feet in front of your nose, and down. As you come out, stretch into Child's Pose.

Date _____

How did you do? Write out your comments about this pose.

_____

Full Locust (Shalabasana)

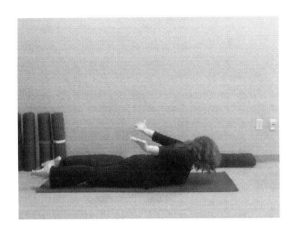

The Full Locust pose strengthens the back muscles and can be challenging so I have listed many modifications below. You begin in a prone position with the weight of your head on your chin or forehead. Arms by your sides, with palms up or palms down (depending on your teachers training, I am not rigid and choose what feels most comfortable for my shoulder joint). Experiment with both techniques and see which way your shoulders are more comfortable. Press your pelvic triangle down. Inhale, lifting your feet and hands. Breathe. People with cardiac problems, back injuries, hernias, recent back or neck surgeries or any abdominal problems should avoid this pose. Your focal point is naturally down and you can counter this with pose with Child's Pose.

Date _____

How did you do? Write out your comments about this pose.

_____

_____

Half Locust (Ardha Shalabasana)

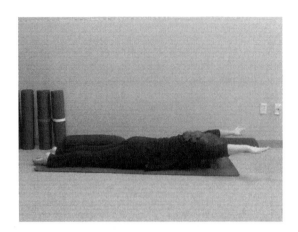

Half Locust is done by leaving your chin, chest and arms on the floor and raise one leg at a time. Or, like the picture above, raise the other half of the body (arms, face and chin) leaving the legs and feet on the floor. This is easier on the lower back. When arms are lifted, reach past your head and really stretch your body long. Children sometimes call this Airplane, leave their legs on the floor and fly their arms all around, out to the sides or front and back.

Date _____

How did you do? Write out your comments about this pose.

_____

_____

Options in the Full Locust (Shalabasana)

Sometimes called Downward Facing Boat

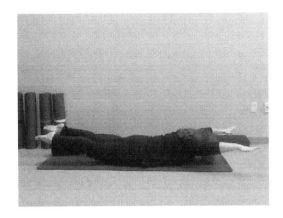

Fly like a Bird

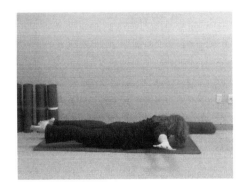

Arms back like an Airplane

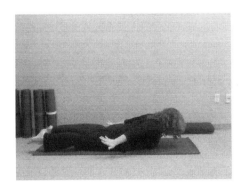

Arms up for Takeoff

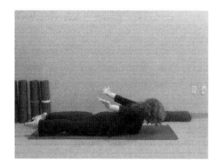

Leave legs on floor

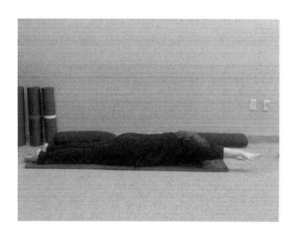

Gentle One Leg King Pigeon Pose (Eka Pada Rajakapotasana)

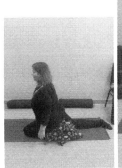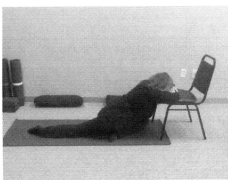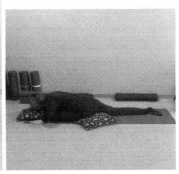

This is a favorite posture for many people with flexible hips. Start in the table pose or down dog pose. Move your left knee up and place it between your hands. Stretch the opposite leg back as you lower your hips. Begin adjusting the front (left) foot out to the side and away from your body so your hips move closer to the floor. Keep your hands grounded and stretch your crown high. There may be a slight back bend. You can also experiment with lowering your forehead to a chair, blocks, pillows or the floor. People who like this pose feel an opening in the hip flexors, thighs, chest and shoulders. If you have knee or hip problems, you may want to skip this pose. Many props can be helpful here: a blanket, pillow, chair or blocks under the hips. Keep your focal point forward or close your eyes to meditate. You can counter this pose by bringing your knees to your chest or any of the seated forward bends.

Date _____

How did you do? Write out your comments about this pose.

_____

_____

Extended Child's Pose (Balasana)

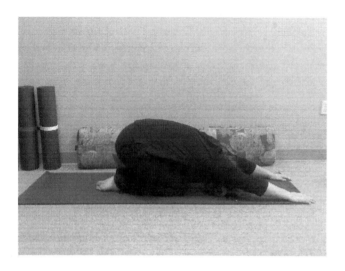

Extended Child's Pose is a resting pose, just like the Classic Child's Pose with your arms stretched out. This can be more comfortable for many people than having the arms wrapped around the body. From kneeling, lean forward, sit back on your heels and rest your chest on your thighs. The weight of your head rests on your forehead. Your arms stretch and extend out in front, reaching. Your knees can be wide, resting the torso in-between your thighs. Close your eyes.

Date _____

How did you do? Write out your comments about this pose.

_____

_____

Restorative Child's Pose (Balasana)

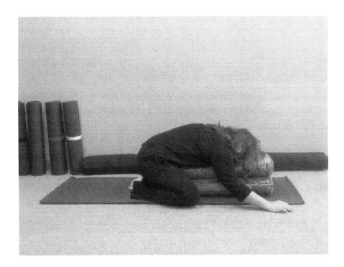

Restorative Child's Pose requires a set up. Put two large bolsters in front of your knees. Your knees will splay out around the bolsters. From kneeling, lean forward, sit back on your heels and rest your chest, face and forehead on the bolsters. The weight of your head should rest on the bolster. Close your eyes.

I have introduced three variations of the Child's Pose, a pose that represents a child in the womb. In an old myth, Krishna lies to his mom about eating mud. When the mom made him open his mouth she saw the whole universe in there. His mom remembers Krishna is divine, even though he is a normal naughty boy sometimes. Children do remind us to be playful and let go of our troubles, or at least put them in perspective. Child's Pose is one we can let go in.

Date _____

How did you do? Write out your comments about this pose.

_____

_____

Gentle Sun Salutation

The Sun Salutation is the centerpiece of many yoga classes. It is a series of common yoga postures linked together with the breath. Some people move fast, some slow. Some do it as a warm up. Some people do 108 of them in a row. There are as many variations of Sun Salutation as there are yogis. People often make up a series of poses that are just for their body type or fitness level. For me, a Sun Salutation is not so much about how many poses you choose to link with the breath, but the linking of the two ideas of strength and surrender. In all Sun Salutations, the poses flow from strong poses with the head up to poses with the face and head down in surrender. Below, I have outlined a gentle version of a classic series. Some people may need a chair for balance as they move through these poses. I have also seen people delete a few poses, so I encourage you to be creative, and adjust the poses to make them as gentle or as challenging as you like.

If you begin to research Sun Salutation on the Internet, you will find what seems to be a million different sequences: classic, sun A, sun B, chair sun salutation, half sun salutations, power sun salutation, and many more. Many teachers will design their own version of the series, adding or subtracting poses. The creativity designing this sequence is unlimited.

Because I teach the poses using the concepts of strength and surrender, it is up to you to let these feelings inform your poses. For example, arms above the head and reaching to the sky may feel strongest for some students while sitting in a chair or wheelchair, but for other students, standing with their feet firmly rooted on a wood floor feels best. This way, each pose in the series is performed and held based on what each student can do safely and comfortably.

My Simple Sun Salutation

Begin in Mountain, arms low, hands to heart center
Arms up to Tall Mountain, add a slight back bend if you choose
Forward fold at the hips, peek the head up with a flat back and with hands next to feet, step back to lunge
Step the other leg back to meet the first
Now you are in plank
Lower yourself to the floor
Choose how far you can push up: Cobra, Sphinx or Upward Facing Dog
Lift hips up to the sky for Downward Facing Dog
Step forward to a lunge, step the other leg up, and now you are in rag doll or forward fold or half forward fold
Lift to Tall Mountain, then lower arms to Mountain, and end with hands at heart center

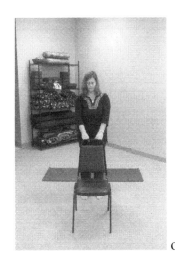 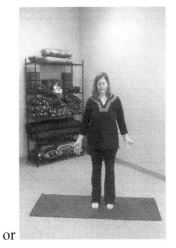
or

Tall Mountain or Raised Hands Pose (Urdhva Hastasana)

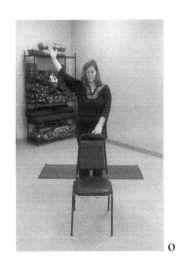 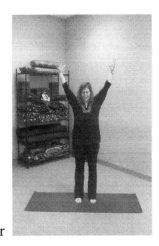
or

Standing Forward Bend (Uttanasana)

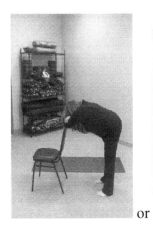 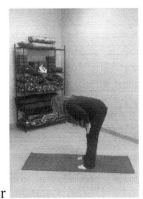 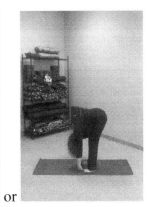
or   or

Low Lunge back (like a Runners Stretch with hands down)

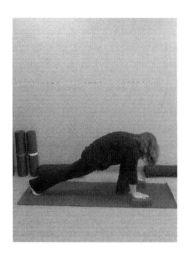

Plank pose

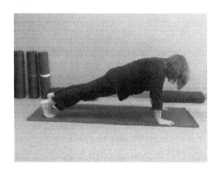

Drop to knees then belly to the floor

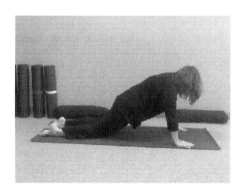

Push up to Cobra or Up Dog

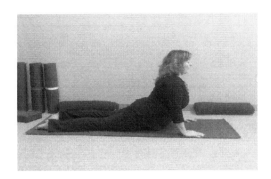

Push hips high up in the air to Down Dog

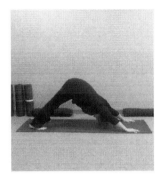

Back into Lunge

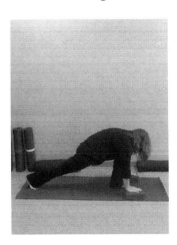

Bring both feet between the hands into a Forward Fold

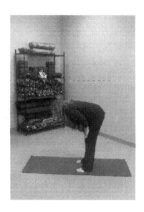

Rise up to your Tall Mountain

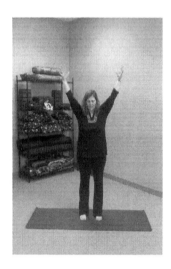

Lower hands to heart center or to your sides in Mountain Pose

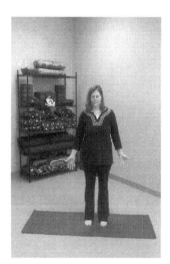

Gentle Seated and Twisting Postures

Seated poses are considered the hardest poses in some schools of yoga because they can be hard on the hips, low back and knees. This is generally why many gentle yoga classes will begin with standing poses, standing balance poses and alternate standing and prone poses in sequences like the sun salutation. Standing and balance poses warm up the large muscles and over time strengthen these, making sitting for long periods less problematic.

The set of poses presented next are seated and twisting poses. In these, the crown of your head is reaching to the sky with the sits bones evenly placed on the mat. Some of these poses are great for meditation and breathing exercises. Just like in other sections, I have presented several poses so you can select which feel safe and comfortable for you. You may need props for a few. These poses lend themselves to slow movements, with plenty of time in the pose and between the poses. All of these poses can be practiced at different levels of difficulty, so every student can experiment, challenge themselves, or back off at any time. As with all the poses common sense precautions are in order.

Easy Seated Pose (Sukhaasana)

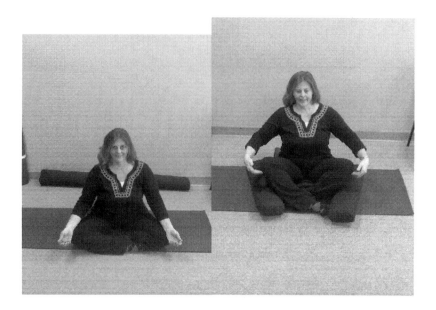

This is a seated cross-legged position on the floor. In Kids Yoga we call it Crisscross Applesauce. Although it is called Easy Seated Pose, it is not easy for many people. Ideally, your spine is straight, your hips are grounded to the floor, your crown is reaching for the sky and your gaze is down or eyes are closed. If it is not easy for you to sit in this position, move to any comfortable position sitting on the floor with your props. Find your own easy seated pose that fits your body. People with knee injuries avoid this exact pose and stretch their legs out. You can use blankets, a block or bolsters under your hips to lift you up and help your knees drop. Your eyes can be closed or looking down and in front.

This is a great pose in which to practice Alternate Nostril Breathing. Bring your hand to your nose and prepare to close off your nostrils using your thumb and middle or ring finger. Close off your left nostril with your finger, then exhale out of the right nostril, inhale in the right nostril and then close off the right with your thumb. Next, exhale through the left nostril and then inhale through the left and then close off the left nostril. Begin again. Alternate Nostril Breathing should not be practiced if you have a cold or a sinus infection, and it should not be practiced too vigorously or too excessively.

Date _____

How did you do? Write out your comments about this pose.

_____

_____

Staff Pose (Dandasana)

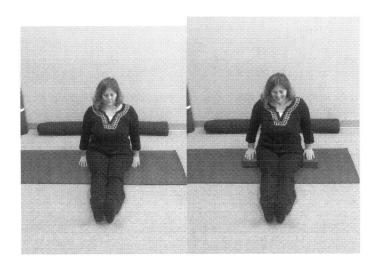

Staff Pose (Dandasana) is the basic seated pose from which all the others originate. Sit on the floor with your legs together. You can sit on a blanket or pillow to lift your pelvis if this is more comfortable. Extend your legs in front of you and flatten your feet. You may get a hamstring stretch so intense it makes you want to stop here. Line your palms up next to your hips and press down into the floor. Reach the crown of your head up to the ceiling. If you have long arms, your hips will lift right up off the floor. If you have short arms, it may be hard to reach the floor, much less press yourself up. If this is the case and you want to lift, put blocks under your palms. Either way, press your heels out and your palms down. This can strengthen the back muscles and improves posture. You may want to avoid this pose, or modify it further, if you have any wrist or lower back trouble. You can place sandbags on your thighs or sit with your back against a wall. Your focal point should be out in front and your gaze down. When you come out of this pose a gentle twist may feel good.

Danda means staff or rod. The story behind the Staff Pose involves the god Krisha holding up a mountain with his pinky finger for seven days of terrible rain. He was protecting the people from the rain, as they were huddled under the mountain. They then used their rods and sticks to help hold up the mountain. The staff also symbolizes the support of the teacher or guru on the yoga path. The more we practice yoga, the more we see teachers all around us and feel gratitude for our teachers, the philosophy and the practice.

Date _____

How did you do? Write out your comments about this pose.

_____

_____

Cow Face Pose (Gomukhasana)

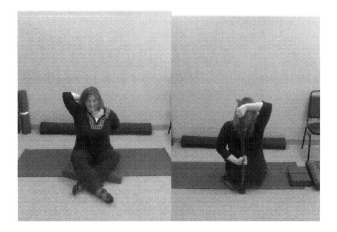

Stay in Easy Seated pose and cross one leg over the opposite ankle or knee. (Or for more challenge cross one leg over and bring your feet back towards your hips.) It can be difficult to cross your legs if your hips are tight, so adjust your legs until you are comfortable. Lift your opposite arm high in the air and drop it down your back, like you are going to scratch your back between your shoulder blades. Reach the other hand around your waist to the back and grab your hands together. If unable to grab hands, reach your fingertips toward each other or hold a strap between your hands. This pose stretches the hips and shoulders at the same time. Rotator cuff and other shoulder problems will not allow this sort of shoulder movement, so adjust the pose for your body. You can also place a blanket under your hips. Your focal point can be in front of your knees on the floor or with your eyes closed. When you come out of the pose, you may want to hug your chest, straighten your legs, or place your feet on the ground, swaying your knees back and forth.

Gomukhasana is called the cow faced pose in English, but the deeper meaning is a bit more subtle. "Go" actually refers to the senses. We can use our senses to help calm the mind. Mukha means a face or facing (mukha is in downward facing dog as well). It also means a passageway, referring to what you are going through. This pose can teach us to be less critical and more accepting of ourselves if the hands do not touch or we cannot cross our legs. Be gentle with yourself and let self-criticism go.

Date _____

How did you do? Write out your comments about this pose.

_____

_____

Gentle Hero Pose (Virasana)

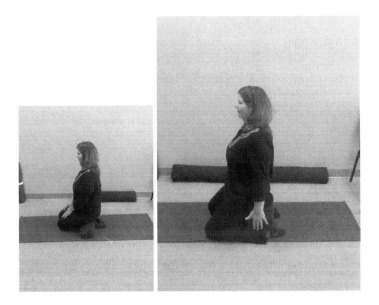

This is an easy seated pose for some people, and impossible for others. Do not even try it if you have major knee problems. From Table Pose, lower your hips back and down to sit on the ground between your feet. You do not have to come all the way down to the ground if that is impossible for you. Very few people in gentle yoga can sit all the way to the ground. Sitting on a block or bolster is more comfortable and perfectly acceptable. Sit tall, back is straight, the crown of your head reaches to the sky. Keep your focus down, in front of your knees, or close your eyes and meditate. To counter this pose, shake your legs out in front of you. Let your feet and legs wobble to and fro.

Hero pose is a good for practicing a breathing technique called Bellows Breath. With your mouth closed, breathe in and out of your nose as fast as possible. Imagine using a little pump to quickly pump up a ball or a tire. Do this about 5 seconds but for no longer than 15 seconds when first starting. Short, fast breaths are used to increase energy. This breath is also called the stimulating breath or rabbit's breath. There is a risk for hyperventilation that can result in loss of consciousness if this exercise is done too much, so try it but don't overdo it.

Date _____

How did you do? Write out your comments about this pose.

Seated Forward Bend (Paschimottanasana)

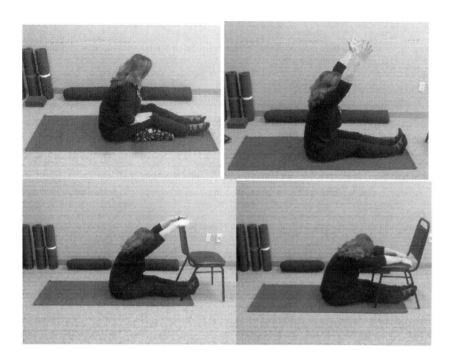

This forward bend with outstretched legs is a favorite for many yogis. Begin in a seated position on the floor, legs extended. Lift your arms overhead. Hinge yourself forward, folding your body in half. Bend forward from your hips and try not to round your back. You can reach your hands to a chair top, chair seat, blocks or, for the very flexible wrap your hands around your feet. Your toes should curl back towards the crown of your head no matter where your hands end up. This provides a deep stretch for entire spine, hamstrings, and calves. If you have had recent or chronic back injury, inflammation, or acute sciatica you will want to avoid this pose. You can place a blanket under your hips and pillows under the knees, keeping your knees as bent as necessary to feel comfortable. Your focal point should be a few feet out in front of your toes or close your eyes and meditate.

Date _____

How did you do? Write out your comments about this pose.

_____

_____

Head to Knee (Janu Sirsasana)

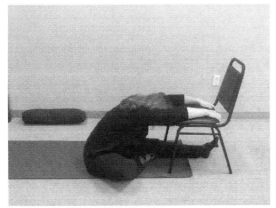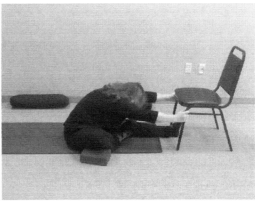

Begin in staff pose. Extend one leg out and place the bottom of the other foot against your inner thigh. Hinge forward from your hips, keeping your back straight. Your hands can reach for a chair, you can rest arms on a chair, or reach toward your toes. Grab your extended foot, calf or thigh. Reach your arms toward your extended foot while the crown of your head stretches toward your toes. Toes should curl back toward the crown of your head, shoulders staying parallel to floor. This pose stretches the calves, hamstring, and lower back. It can calm menstrual or menopausal discomfort as well as the overall nervous system. You may want to avoid this pose if you have low blood pressure, knee injury, asthma, or chronic back problems. Your focal point will probably be at your shins. Knees to chest, is a good counter pose.

Date _____

How did you do? Write out your comments about this pose.

_____

_____

Bound Angle (Baddha Konasana)

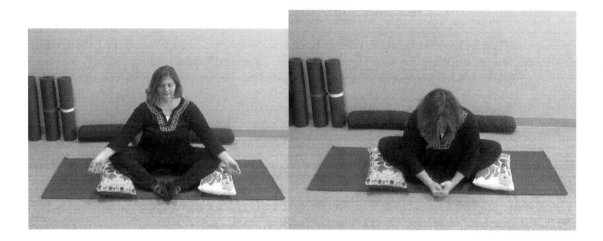

Begin in an easy seated pose on the floor. Lift your hips on to a blanket if your hips are tight. Put the soles of your feet together and slowly drop your knees out to the sides. If your knees stay high, you can prop them up for comfort using rolled up blankets, pillows or bolsters. Keep the edges of your feet on the floor. Your knees will rest and relax onto the props. Reach the crown of your head to the sky and if you choose, you can bend forward from your hips, kissing the toes. This pose is said to stimulate the abdominal organs, ovaries, prostate gland, bladder, and kidneys. You can feel the stretch to your inner thighs, groins, and knees. You may choose to avoid this pose if you have knee or hip trouble. Your focal point should be somewhere past your toes. Any of the seated twists or forward bends will be good counter poses when coming out of Bound Angle.

Some of my students and teacher trainees tell me: "I do not like meditation", "they did not teach meditation in my teacher training", "my mind will not stop running", "I cannot sit still", "I can't meditate more than one second", "I do not know how to meditate" and "meditation is too hard". I was taught that the yoga postures were designed to assist and prepare you for meditation. All of the first postures written about in yoga texts were various ways to sit for meditation. Give it a try. Find a comfortable seated posture and learn how to meditate like the sages of old.

Date _____

How did you do? Write out your comments about this pose.

_____

_____

72

Progressive Seated Twist (Ardha Matsyendrasana I, II, III)

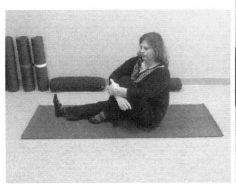 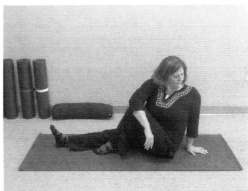

Begin seated on the floor in Dandasana. In stage 1, bring one knee up and line that foot with the knee on the floor. Twist your chest toward your bent knee. You can hold the knee, wrap your arm around the knee or even twist so the arm moves past the upper knee. In stage 2, we change the leg position. Begin with one leg straight out, cross the other leg over the grounded leg and place that foot on floor close to your knee. Some people can move to stage 3 by also bending the grounded leg and placing both feet near the hips. The whole bottom should stay grounded on the floor in each stage. Twists stretch the spine and stimulate the digestive system. People with recent or chronic knee, hip, back or shoulder injury may want to avoid these types of postures. Place a cushion under your hips or a block under the hand behind your back to simplify the pose. Your eyes can follow around with the twist and gaze over your shoulder to protect the neck from cranking too much. Twist the other direction to counter the pose.

Date _____

How did you do? Write out your comments about this pose.

_____

Seated Wide Angle Forward Bend (Upavistha Konasana)

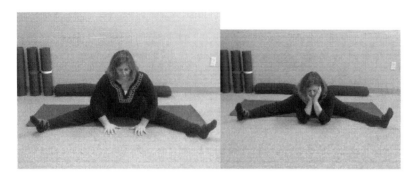

This is a seated forward bend with the legs outstretched wide. Begin in any seated floor position and extend your legs as wide apart as is comfortable for you. Begin to walk your hands out between your legs slowly, while hinging from the hips. Walk the hands back and sit tall. Try it again and walk your hands out a little further. Go as far as feels comfortable and stop. Your hands may be on the floor or grabbing your legs, ankles, or toes. Keep a flat back. You will feel a stretch up the spine, hamstrings, and calves. It is not a pose for those with recent or chronic back injury, inflammation, or acute sciatica. You can place a firm blanket under your hips and bend your knees to feel comfortable. Your eyes can rest a few feet out in front. A counter pose is Knees to Chest.

Date _____

How did you do? Write out your comments about this pose.

_____

Upward Boat (Navasana)

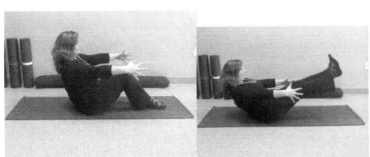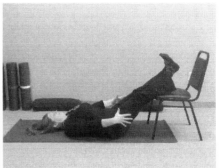

Begin in a seated position with your back straight, knees up, hands under your knees or behind the thighs for support. Hold both legs and lift one off the floor. Set it down and lift the other. Set it down and lift both feet up off the floor for a few inches. Experiment with letting your hands go and then putting them back. Rest. Slowly lift one leg and then the other. Let your hands float out to the side and then toward your knees. This is serious core work and many people in gentle yoga will keep one foot on the ground. This posture strengthens abdominal muscles. You must be very careful not to strain your neck. If you have any injury to your abdomen, neck, back, or hips, you may choose to skip this one. This posture can be done with your forearms down or by lowering the entire back to the floor and just lifting your legs. You can also place your feet on a chair or the wall to practice. Your focal point should be straight ahead in front of you. You can counter this pose with Knees to Chest or gentle twists.

Date _____

How did you do? Write out your comments about this pose.

Gentle Supine Poses and Backbends

My field, psychology, seems especially connected to yoga, as both are so focused on mental processes and behavior. One of the most interesting psychologists, Carl G. Jung, was an artist and an analyst extraordinaire. His style of analysis was to explore the mysterious unconscious, teach people how to access it, and view it as a form of language revealed through symbols and myths. He viewed these symbols as communication, unfolding and revealing an important message to healing and wholeness. Jung may say something is being pulled forth from the individual subconscious when symbols come up, dreams for the future, things not done. So many of the yoga postures I have presented in this book are rooted in and connected to myths and folklore. I do not believe there is any perfect way to do a posture, only the way the posture works for your body and when right for you, allowing it to communicate with your mysterious unconscious.

The set of supine poses will allow for that communication. The poses presented in this final section are gentle backbends and poses done flat on the back, Most of these become restorative yoga poses in a gentle yoga class and some are great for practicing yogic meditation. Many people will become so relaxed in these poses they will experience their first glimpses of a very peaceful mediation. Just like in the prior sections I have presented a variety of poses and you select which feel safe and comfortable for you. I use many props with these poses and move very slowly from one to another. You may want to spend longer in these poses but do not fall asleep. As in the other sections, all these poses can be practiced at a few levels of difficulty so every student can experiment, challenge or back off at any time.

Knees to Chest (Apanasana)

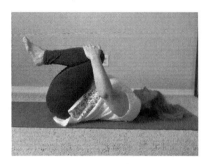

You may want to set up your space with a thick mat or blanket under your body for this pose. Begin flat on your back and simply lift the knees to your chest or as close as you can get them. Wrap arms around your legs below the knees, holding on to opposite elbows, forearms, wrists or fingers. Your knees can also be placed out to the side of your rib cage. Tuck your chin into the chest with head flat on floor. Press your sacrum into floor. Feel the length of your whole spine press into floor. Relax legs, feet and hips. Breathe. The focal point is on the ceiling or eyes closed. You can counter this pose with the Corpse pose.

From Corpse Pose practice the 3-Part Breath (or Dirga Pranayama). Sometimes I call this the sniff, sniff, sniff breath. You breathe into the lowest lobe of the lung, then inhale a little more air which fills the middle lobe of the lung and inhale a little more which fills the top lobe. You feel really full of air and want to exhale but in a controlled way exhale from top of the lungs to the bottom. The idea of the three part breath is to experience filling up the entire lungs and exhaling fully to empty the lungs. When you trick the body into full exhale like this a deep inhale follows. This breath promotes good sleep and reduces physical discomforts. A full yogic breath is also called Mahat Yoga Pranayama.

Date _____

How did you do? Write out your comments about this pose.

Reclining Big Toe (Supta Padangusthasana)

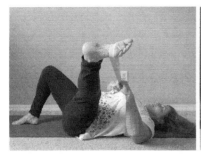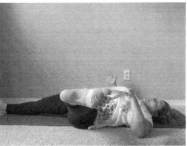

As you can see this is the same pose as one of our balancing poses, we have just changed the orientation and do the pose flat on the back. Begin on your back, bend one knee and grab that toe. If you can't reach your toes grab your ankle or shin. Stretch that leg out, bring it back and think about how this feels in your hips, knees and ankles. If you can, stretch your leg out as far as you can go and hold for a few deep ocean sounding breaths. This pose will stretch your hips, thighs, hamstrings, and calves. If you have recent injury or inflammation to the legs, shoulders, or neck, you may choose to avoid this pose. If you have trouble grabbing your toe and have a strap handy, you can slip the strap over the ball of your out stretched foot and add many inches to your reach. You can do this pose with the heel resting against a wall as well. Your focal point will be the ceiling or close your eyes. You can counter this pose with a gentle twist.

Date _____

How did you do? Write out your comments about this pose.

_____

Reclining Bound Angle (Supta Badda Konasana)

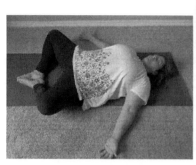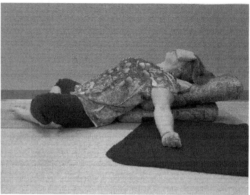

As you can see this pose is the same as a seated pose, Bound Angle, but the orientation has changed. Begin on your back and move the soles of your feet together, flopping the knees out to the sides. Relax the rest of the body comfortably, arms resting to the sides with palms up. Breathe. To rest even deeper use bolsters under the knees for support and do not bring the knees down too far. You also can use blankets, pillows or blocks under knees, a belt supporting the hips, and blankets to cover up so you do not get chilly. Many of my students like to do final relaxation in this pose. Avoid the pose if you have a groin or knee problems.

This posture is a favorite to practice the fifth limb of yoga (pratyahara). This is typically defined as the process of withdrawing the mind from sensory impressions (taste, touch, sight, hearing and smell). Another view of the fifth limb is the transcending of, rather than the withdrawing from, sensory impressions. Either way, we get away from our personal distractions and we are moved to deep relaxation. Common techniques for the fifth limb of yoga are guided meditation, body scan meditation, squeezing and relaxing the body parts in a particular order, and other techniques that result in a mind that is undisturbed by everything going on around it.

Date _____

How did you do? Write out your comments about this pose.

_____

_____

Supine Spinal Twist (Jathara Parivartanasana)

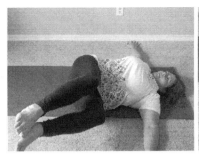 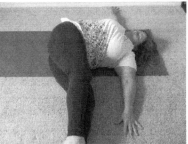 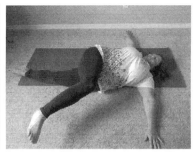

Begin on your back and stretch your arms out to a "T". Draw your knees towards your chest and then drop both knees to one side and let them stop when it feels like enough of a twist. Relax into the posture. If knees come to floor, experiment with straightening the legs out. Breathe. This pose stretches the back and abdominal muscles so make sure you feel comfortable as you hold this pose. You can keep your knees bent and just roll them from one side to the other. Or bend one knee to chest and drop this one over the opposite hip for a one leg spinal twist. Keep your eyes closed.

Date _____

How did you do? Write out your comments about this pose.

81

Gentle Fish (Matsyasana)

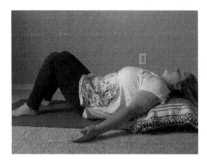

In one ancient yoga myth, a nosey fish (matsya) eavesdrops on the god Shiva talking to his lover, Parvati, about yoga. The fish becomes completely enlightened and realizes Shiva is the first guru (teacher) and the fish is the first yoga student.

For this propped up version of the pose you may want to prep your space before you lie down. Place 2-3 folded blankets under your upper back to support this pose and make sure your head is resting on blankets. Begin on your back, fully supported by the blankets, with your arms alongside your body and your legs a few inches apart. Slide your hands (palms down) under your thighs, or tuck just your elbows under your body. Your head and neck are supported and if you need more support, add a small neck pillow. There should be no weight on the top of the head. Breathe. Be careful or avoid this pose if you have any chronic arm, shoulder, neck or back problems. Keep your eyes closed. You can counter this pose with the Knees to Chest pose.

Date _____

How did you do? Write out your comments about this pose.

Bridge and Supported Bridge (Setu Banda Sarvangasana)

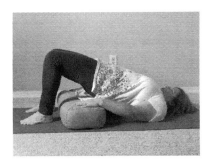

This is another pose you begin on your back, but this time keep your knees high and your feet on the floor under your knees. Slide your hands (palms down) under your hips or rest hands alongside hips. Lift the hips as far as feels comfortable, this may be a few inches or much more. Keep the soles of your feet flat on the floor. Make sure your head, shoulders and neck are comfortable and resting on the ground naturally, not arched. Just the hips have moved up off the ground. Keep the eyes closed and relax. Come down whenever you like and you can counter this pose with the Knees to Chest pose.

A restorative bridge pose requires a yoga prop such as blankets, flat bolsters or a block to place under your hips. If you would like to try this pose, as you lift your hips slide the prop under your hips, or have a partner do if for you. The idea is to get a lift from the props under the hips and let the props support the posture without using any effort. Make sure your head, shoulders and neck are comfortable and resting on the ground naturally and come down off the prop carefully.

Date _____

How did you do? Write out your comments about this pose.

Gentle Inversions

When I was in my 20s, I lived in a country thousands of miles from home in an Indian neighborhood. My sweet landlord brought me to a yoga class down the street taught by a tiny Indian woman in her empty living room. We paid her $1 or $2 per yoga class, which I believe was her only income. She was a wonderful yoga teacher, and taught me how to stand on my head properly for the first time, but her main focus with us was discipline. My class mates rarely did any postures, they liked to gossip and drink tea. They talked quite a lot about husbands, arranged marriages, and always asked how many marriage proposals I received at the bus stop that day. Our teacher would get frustrated and yell "Look at Beth, she is so big but she still does all the postures. Put your tea down." It may have been one of my favorite yoga classes of all time. This teacher understood what we did not yet, that yoga really did require getting your mind off all the exciting things going on and trying to focus.

More and more teachers are getting away from teaching inversions in a group class, but stick to private lessons for inversions. They can take a lot of time to master. I no longer practice the following poses: full shoulder stand, plow, headstand or handstand. Why? Because they hurt my neck. Many people in gentle yoga have neck and back problems and there are other inversions we can do such as those described over the next few pages. In some of my classes we practice: Happy Baby, Dead Bug, Half Shoulder Stand and Legs up the Wall. You will notice as you read through these pose descriptions the neck stays supported by the floor. These gentle inversions change the orientation we are used to (head up) and yet they are gentle and easy to learn. And all these inversions prepare us for meditation.

Happy Baby (Ananda Balasana)

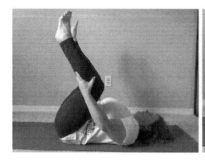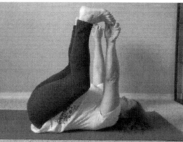

Lying on floor stretch your legs toward the sky and bend the knees. See if you can grab your toes, feet, ankles, calves or the back of the knees. Where ever your hands land, hold the pose and breathe. Close your eyes and relax your head, neck and shoulders. Hold this for a few breaths. Imagine you are a happy baby in your crib and smile. Release the pose and rest on the floor.

Patanjali's Yoga Sutras discusses the peace a person can have by joining the busy, thinking mind with cosmic intelligence. These sutras serve as a reference guide to yogis everywhere. I like one translation of the first sutra "NOW we begin the practice of yoga" reminding me to approach each day and each pose with fresh eyes.

Date _____

How did you do? Write out your comments about this pose.

Dead Bug (Matkunasana)

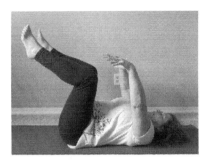

The Sanskrit means bug pose, or bed bug pose, depending on the dictionary, but people do call it Dead Bug Pose. The pose is similar to Happy Baby and some people like it better. Lying on floor, stretch your arms and legs toward the sky. Bend your knees and elbows a bit for comfort. Hold and breathe. Close your eyes and relax your head, neck and shoulders. Hold this for a few breaths or more.

Patanjali's second yoga sutra is said to be the first definition of yoga. There are many translations as to what it really means but this sutra defines yoga as the complete settling of the activity of the mind or the joining together of two things that have never been separate.

Date _____

How did you do? Write out your comments about this pose.

_____

_____

Half Shoulder Stand (Arha Salamba Sarvangasana)

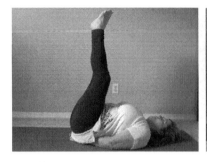 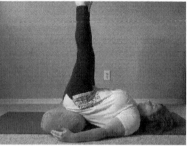

Lying on floor with arms at the sides of the body, bend your knees, tuck them to your chest and place your hips in your hands. Your hands can hold your hips for support or your hips can stay grounded. Raise your feet up in the air a bit. You can keep your knees straight, bent or even keep your knees closer to your chest. No weight should be on neck or head, this is a movement lifting the legs. Avoid this pose all together if you have serious back or neck problems, eye problems like glaucoma (avoid inversions with eye problems), brain injury or surgery, blood pressure instability, or pregnancy.

In the limbs of yoga the fourth and fifth (breathing and withdrawing the senses) are bridges to meditation. We do these all the time as we practice the poses. Limb six, dharana, begins to nudge you off the bridge by using an object of meditation. The object of meditation should be something you can see or feel. The discipline is trying to stay focused on it. This is just a place to start, but even with simple techniques one can build concentration with practice. In each of the poses you can settle your mind on one thing, your choice, for any extended period of time.

Date _____

How did you do? Write out your comments about this pose.

_____

_____

Legs up the Wall (Viparita Karani)

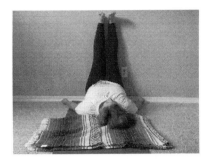

There are a few ways to move into this pose. I sit on the floor with my side and hip next to the wall. As you lean back to the floor, rotate your bottom to the wall and slide the legs up the wall. Adjust your bottom to your comfort either touch the wall or a little bit away from the wall. The back of the leg will be up against the wall. Some people will just have heels touching the wall. This position allows for a reverse of blood flow in the body to relieve strain, calm the mind, stretches the legs, relieves leg pain. To modify this bend your knees and maybe even put the soles of your feet together. Some people will place a bolster or stacked blankets under their hips, but I do not find that comfortable. Pad under your head and neck with a flat blanket so your head is not on a hard floor. Your focal point can be on the ceiling or eyes closed with an eye pillow.

I took a yoga class once that always began with 15 minutes in this pose. The students were very successful, driven and stressed. My old yoga teacher may have chosen to begin class with legs up the wall pose because in this flipped over position you have to let go and surrender. It is a bit harder to worry about things.

Date _____

How did you do? Write out your comments about this pose.

Relaxation or Corpse Pose (Savasana)

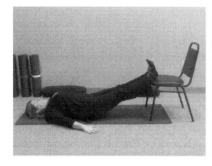 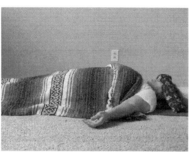

Our final pose in gentle yoga is Savasana, also known as corpse pose or the relaxation pose. This is considered the hardest pose in yoga because in this pose we are to completely relax every part of our mind and body. Begin on your back and move your arms to side of the body with palms up about 8 inches from your torso. Your legs will rest about a foot apart, with your feet falling out to the sides. Close your eyes and breathe softly. This pose is not for people who cannot easily get up and down from the floor, and in this case we do the relaxation in a chair. Many people will place a bolster or blanket under the knees or cover their body with towel or blanket to be more comfortable. The use of a towel over the eyes or an eye pillow will help by cutting down on the light. Moving out of this deep relaxation pose should be done slowly with care, ending in the Easy Seated Pose for meditation.

While in the pose you may want to try the ancient process of meditation called Yoga Nidra. This is a specific guided meditation which induces physical, mental and emotional relaxation. Nidra translates to "sleep" so Yoga Nidra is sometimes called "Yoga Sleep." Experts in the process report deep healing happens in this state. This guided meditation will help you understand the mind portion of our body-mind practice.

Date _____

How did you do? Write out your comments about this pose.

_____

_____

Gentle Conclusion

As you read through these pages I hope you discovered the huge variety of ways you can make the practice of yoga your own. Simple adjustments, modifications and the use of props change the practice from intimidating to easy. The main benefit to making this practice of postures easy on your body is the deep relaxation and peace you experience. From here you will have a much easier time practicing all the meditation techniques so central to the yoga system. Yoga has been a personal development system for millions of people throughout history and there is no reason to be intimidated. These gentle poses will empower you to make this system part of your lifestyle.

When I began taking yoga classes in the early 1980s every type of body was included. I never once thought yoga was only for skinny, flexible, young women because my classes were very diverse. All my teachers were over 40. I remember a class where it seemed I was surrounded by men, all of us struggling with our flexibility, so I never thought it was just a girl thing. No one seemed particularly thin or lovely when I look back to my first classes. I was barely twenty and saw plenty of grey hair. I also studied yoga when I lived overseas and it seemed everyone was encouraged and included if they showed an interest. We did not have mats, we used towels. We had no fancy clothes, just something modest we could move in. There were no props, or straps or pillows although I could have used a few. I remember one of the reasons I was so comfortable in yoga class was because it was so inclusive and diverse.

After practicing yoga through the decades of my life (seriously and just for fun) I am convinced some of the benefits of yoga you read about in medical journals and the popular press have more to do with practicing the entire eight limb system than just a simple set of physical postures. This includes the social disciplines, getting along with others and enjoying a peaceful life. Letting go, humility and an acceptance of what cannot be changed are part of the practice. Also, personal disciplines like willpower, study and commitment are practices we take off the mat and into our daily life at school, work and home. The physical postures, with all their myth and folklore, are only one eighth of the practice. The breathing techniques, which I have touched on as well, are physical in nature but begin to assist the mind to settle down and prepare for deeper meditation. Breathing relaxes us and we do have some control over our breath. All the meditation techniques in yoga help us transcend the ordinary problems in life. Being with like-minded people is excellent for your health. Living a peaceful, stress free, simple lifestyle cannot hurt. All of it together is more powerful than just one piece of it and I predict researchers of the yogic system will continue to examine all of it.

Example Posture Sequences

Warm Up:
Self-care is your assignment

← Inspiration
Teacher
Healer
Artist

Pull out the essence

Essence - communicating to groups

Gentle Posture Series 1

Seated Center with Ocean (Ujjayi) Breath
10 minute Warm up on floor (on back knees, ankles, toes, hip circles, reverse pigeon, structural warm up for the neck)
Table
Cat
Cow
Down Dog
Rag doll
Mountain (Tadasana)
Crescent Moon
Standing backbend
Standing forward
Warrior 1 & 2
Mountain
Half Sun Salute A (stay on floor)
Cobra - 3 stages, Chest, rib cage, navel
Child's Pose
Bound Angle
Seated Twist
Upward boat
Bridge
Knees to Chest
Legs up wall
1/2 knee to chest
Supine spinal twist
Relaxation

Gentle Posture Series 2

Seated Center with Ujjayi Breath
Full warm up

Table
Down Dog
Move up to standing
Mountain Pose
Ujjayi Breath
Warm up shoulders
Crescent Moon
Standing Backbend
Standing Forward Bend
Warrior 1 & 2
Triangle
Tadasana
Sun Salutation
Down Dog
Cobra - 3 stages, your choice
Locust
Child's Pose
Bound Angle
Seated Twist - Stages 1,2 & 3, your choice
Upward Boat

Bridge
Knees to Chest
Legs up wall
1/2 Knee to Chest
Supine Spinal Twist
Supine Tree
Supine Bound Angle

Savasana

Gentle Yoga Posture Series 3

Warm up
Table
Cat
Cow
Plank
Down Dog
Rag doll up
Tadasana
Crescent moon
Standing backbend
Standing forward
Chair
Warrior 1 & 2, extended triangle, triangle (then other side)
Tadasana
Sun Salute A
Half sun salute and rest on the ground.
Practice sphinx as modification to cobra.
Cobra - 3 stages, Chest, rib cage, navel.
Airplane
Child's pose
Hero, yoga arms out, up, behind
Wide leg stretch
Legs together
Head to knees/ankles
Bound Angle
Seated Twist
Upward Boat
Bridge
Both Knees to Chest
Legs up the wall
1/2 Knee to Chest
Supine Spinal Twist
Savasana
Yoga Nidra

Gentle Yoga Posture Series 4

Each pose is 5 or more breaths

Centering and Breathing

Sun Salute A
Chair
Triangle
Revolved Triangle Pose
Warrior 1 & 2

Extended Side Angle Pose
Pyramid Pose

Half Moon Pose
Dancer Pose

Eagle
Tree

Down Dog
Upward Facing Dog
Locust Pose

Cow Face Pose
Boat Pose
Hero Pose
Pigeon Pose

Fish Pose

Half Shoulder Stand
Savasana

Gentle Yoga Posture Series 5

Gentle Warm Ups

Mountain
Tall Mountain
Crescent Moon
Mountain

Half Forward Bend
Rag Doll
Mountain
Mini Back Bend

Wide Angle Forward Bend
Walk hands left to right
5 pointed Star

Warrior 1
Reverse Warrior
Plank
Down Dog
Up Dog
Child Pose

Table Pose
Cat
Cow
Sphinx
Cobra

Staff Pose
Boat Pose
Seated Twist

Knees to Chest
Happy Baby
Dead Bug

Legs up the Wall

Savasana

About the Author

Beth Daugherty, M.S., M.A., E-RYT, RCYT

Beth is the founder of Lifespan Yoga®, Director of Teacher Training, and author of the Lifespan Yoga® Books. She has lived in three different yoga centers and trained with a variety of teachers since the early 1980s. Visit www.LifespanYoga.com for more information and check out Beth's other books on www.Amazon.com:

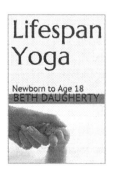

Lifespan Yoga®: Developmental Psychology Meets the Practice and Teaching of Yoga (2014) is for those interested in yoga for children and teens, from newborns to age 18. I highlight the connection between modern research and the eight limbs of yoga in each of the developmental stages children go through. This is written for parents who love yoga and yoga teachers who love children.

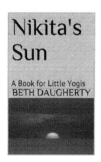

Nikita's Sun (2012) is a children's story I wrote for one of my little students who was learning the Sun Salutation in Kids Yoga.

Sign up for Beth's newsletter at www.LifespanYoga.com

Made in the USA
Charleston, SC
29 July 2015